THE
BROWN FAT
REVOLUTION

THE BROWN FAT REVOLUTION

TRIGGER YOUR BODY'S GOOD FAT

TO LOSE WEIGHT AND BE HEALTHIER

JAMES R. LYONS, M.D.

ST. MARTIN'S PRESS ❧ NEW YORK

This book is intended as a reference volume only, not as a medical manual. The information given here is designed to help you make informed decisions about your health. The exercise and dietary programs in this book are not intended as a substitute for any exercise routine or dietary regimen that may have been prescribed by your doctor. As with all exercise and dietary programs, you should get your doctor's permission before beginning.

The information in this book is meant to supplement, not replace, proper exercise training. All forms of exercise pose some inherent risks. The editor and publisher advise readers to take full responsibility for their safety and know their limits. If you suspect that you have a medical problem, we urge you to seek competent medical help.

Photographs by Deborah Feingold Photography
Book design by Gretchen Achilles

www.stmartins.com

Library of Congress Cataloging-in-Publication Data

Lyons, James R.
    The brown fat revolution : trigger your body's good fat to lose weight and be healthier / James R. Lyons.—1st ed.
        p. cm
    ISBN 978-0-312-59540-1
    1. Weight loss. 2. Brown adipose tissue. 3. Fat cells. I. Title.
RM222.2 .L96 2009
613.2'5 —dc22

2009019890

First Edition: September 2009

10 9 8 7 6 5 4 3 2 1

THIS BOOK IS DEDICATED TO PENNY,
"MY GIRL" SINCE AGE NINE!

CONTENTS

ACKNOWLEDGMENTS

My amazing children, Brooke, Blake, and Chloe, for their respect and genuine enthusiasm. Thank you, Brooke, for your meticulous early edits; Blake for your inspiring artistic contributions; and Chloe for your intuitive opinions of the market. The late Elena Lyons, my mom, for aligning the stars for me. I feel her influence every day.

I would like to thank my patients. Your trust and hard work allowed me to develop *The Brown Fat Revolution* nutrition and fitness programs to help each of you look your absolute best.

Eileen Cope, you are amazing! Without you, this book would not have happened. Thank you for two years of "working it out" with me and then brilliantly framing the concepts to produce *The Brown Fat Revolution*. Your ability to connect the right people at the right time is simply magical.

Kathy Huck for your masterful editing and enthusiastic interest in *The Brown Fat Revolution*. No one could have organized the principles better than you.

Sally Richardson at St. Martin's Press for seeing the importance of *Brown Fat* from the start. Your acknowledgment of my ideas was a major turning point in this project.

George Witte at St. Martin's for the opportunity to do this book.

John J. Murphy, Ann Day, and Tara Cibelli at St. Martin's for making this experience an exciting one.

Karen Moline for your brilliant words. Your ability to connect to my thoughts and put them on paper was phenomenal. The passion you bring to your work is exhilarating. I look forward to our future collaborations.

Robert Gottlieb for recognizing the importance of "brown fat" from the very beginning and bringing me on board at Trident Media.

Maggie Robinson for your fresh approach to eating.

Cathy Cash for connecting me to Robert and Eileen.

Kathy Roberts, my assistant, for everything.

Rick Carbone for convincing me that it was okay to take time out for my own body.

Ken Wallach for your brilliant training and fitness ideas.

Christopher (Topher) Tornow for your personal training.

Alyse Diamond at St. Martin's Press.

Alexandra for being so courteous and always making contact with Eileen so effortless.

Deborah Feingold for your artistry. You turned a tedious experience into fun.

Sara Branch, copy editor, for your meticulous attention to detail.

Dr. Bill Little for your incredible work on volume and the "devolving" face. Your words caused my epiphany on aging and fat distribution.

The "olympic level" surgical team: Dr. Robert Ljungquist, Dr. John Mc-Carthy, Paula Martinka, R.N., and Pat Cobb, R.N. Thanks for making my Thursdays so efficient and for listening to my incessant discussion of brown and yellow fat.

Nancy Hancock for your long friendship and respect. They mean a great deal to me.

Ivyeyesediting.com for the incredible assistance with the first proposal.

Dolores Guarino, R.N., for eighteen years of incredible support. It is not forgotten.

THE
BROWN FAT
REVOLUTION

INTRODUCTION

Let me tell you a story about fat.

"Have you ever seen such a thing?" asked my patient Lisa as she came in for an appointment one rainy day several years ago. "It's worse than when I was pregnant. At least then I had a baby inside. But look at me now. This is just *gross!*"

Lisa was sweet, sassy—and seriously desperate. With one swift glance I immediately understood why. At the age of fifty-one, she was burdened with an absolutely enormous floppy and lumpy fold of belly fat. She patted it and grimaced as she shifted uncomfortably in her chair.

"Don't worry, I have seen such a thing," I told her, and she visibly relaxed in relief. "So many times before, in fact, that there's a name for it: a panniculus. It's caused by the kind of fat in your body that's yellow and unhealthy. I call it McDonald's fat."

"I don't care if you call it Burger King fat or Wendy's fat!" she joked. "Just get rid of it, *please!*"

Because Lisa's panniculus was so disproportionate to the rest of her petite frame, her only option, unlike for most of my patients, was a drastic one, and we scheduled a tummy tuck.

On the day of her surgery, after I made my initial incision, the surgical residents and the anesthesiologist watched benignly, expecting yet another routine procedure. Then they peered over at Lisa's abdomen, and I heard them gasp aloud.

"I have *never* seen anything like that before," the anesthesiologist told me, his eyes round with shock over his surgical mask as he looked at the mounds of bright yellow fat in Lisa's abdomen. As I explained what it was, you could have heard a pin drop in that surgical suite.

The more I explained the difference between Lisa's yellow fat and the good kind of brown fat that makes a body look and feel healthy and vibrant, the more I realized how many misperceptions there are about fat—even in the well-educated medical community.

Contrary to popular belief, you see, fat is the key to a nice flat belly. And *fat* is the key to a youthful-looking face and body, as well.

But here's the crucial element to unlocking the power of fat. *Not all fat is the same*. The fat that keeps you looking and feeling vibrant is not the unhealthy old, soft, and mushy yellow fat like the astonishing amount (*ten* pounds!) I plucked out of Lisa during her operation. I can tell you from my decades of surgical experience that there is a fat that is healthy and highly desirable. It is what I call brown fat. Brown fat is firm and resilient and gives our bodies a youthful shape—it keeps our cheeks round and our butts in place.

This book will prove to you that once you understand the difference between brown fat and yellow fat, you can make the changes in how you eat and how you move to get rid of the bad and replace it with the good, no matter what your age.

The Brown Fat Revolution is the first book to show you how to use your own fat to dramatically rejuvenate your face and body.

VOLUME = GOOD BROWN FAT = YOUTH

When you hear the words "plastic surgeon," what immediately comes to mind? If you're like many consumers, you probably think about something like face-lifts or liposuction or even a television show like *Extreme Makeover*.

As a plastic surgeon, I've realized that it takes a lot more than just expensive surgery for my patients to achieve the best results they're hoping for. I've spent my entire professional life looking at shape and contour, coupling this knowledge with a firm understanding of science and physiology so I can do the best job possible, moving fat around to create beauty and youth in the face and body.

As a physician, I've studied nutrition and metabolic functions for over three decades. And as a bodybuilder for more than two decades, I've learned how to literally confuse my metabolism so that my muscles continue to strengthen even while fat is never deposited in my body.

I've also had many years of experience listening to women's hopes and needs, learning to understand them better so I can help them look and feel the best they possibly can. What I hear, over and over again, from these patients are statements like "I'm eating the same and exercising the same way as I've done for the last twenty years, but my waist just keeps getting bigger," or "I don't look the way I feel inside. In fact, I'm starting to look like my mother."

I tell them that all the money in the world can buy you as many medical procedures as you want, but it can never buy you a truly healthy, beautiful body.

I also tell them that, without question, the most important anti-aging concept for me is the *language of volume*. (All plastic surgery stems from this notion, as the Greek word *plastikos* means "to shape.")

It's volume that gives faces their youthful contours and soft curves. It's volume that makes us look young and rounded.

And it's good brown fat that gives you the volume you want, in the places you want it!

Brown fat is typical of youthful curves and excellent nutrition and health. Yellow fat is typical of age and poor nutrition; it creates the characteristic face and body shapes that we associate with aging, such as a round lower abdomen, jiggly arms, and soft, enlarged breasts.

That there is such a noticeable difference between brown fat and yellow fat was highlighted in a front-page article by science reporter Gina Kolata, published in *The New York Times* on April 8, 2009, entitled "Calorie-Burning Fat? Studies Say You Have It." This article discussed the results of several different research studies, whose results were published in the *New England Journal of Medicine* (360, no. 15 [2009]: 1500–1508), that scientifically documented the role of brown fat cells. These studies concentrated on the thermogenic, or heat-burning, properties of brown fat found deep in the body. This type of brown fat was previously thought to be vestigial in adult humans; it had been thought to control temperature only in small mammals and infants. The conclusions of the studies were not only that there are different types of fat in the body, but that deep brown fat can burn more calories than yellow fat, particularly when triggered by cold temperatures.

Researchers were elated by these findings, as the hope is that eventually some completely new form of weight-loss drug may be developed—tackling excess fat *internally*, on a cellular level, by stimulating these thermogenic properties of deep brown fat, rather than by tackling caloric consumption.

And I was elated because these studies were a strictly controlled, scientific validation of three of my clinical impressions: that there are different types of fat in the body; that the more brown fat you have, the leaner you tend to be; and that different types of fat can be modulated by lifestyle, diet, and exercise so that you can convert yellow fat into brown fat.

These findings are thrilling if not revolutionary for those who study and work with fat, as they further our understanding of what fat is—that there is a spectrum of fat in the body, that different kinds of fat have different properties, and that aspects of our behavior (diet, exercise, medications) can affect our fat stores.

These studies concentrated on studying deep brown fat under the microscope at the cellular level, specifically on stimulating certain brown fat cells in the neck, upper back, and along the spine to regulate energy metabolism. These fat cells contain high concentrations of mitochondria, the energy boosters of the cells. The mitochondria ramp up the metabolism of these fat cells, and the iron they contain gives the fat cells their brown hue.

I, on the other hand, have spent nearly thirty years working with thousands of bodies, during which time I've learned that not all skin is the same—and not all fat is, either. I see this every time I perform any surgical procedure. The brown fat that I see appears throughout the body, usually in the subcutaneous plane (immediately below the skin's surface). This subcutaneous brown fat gets its distinctive hue due to the dense network of connective tissue and blood vessels coursing through its well-proportioned fat cells, making it light brown or tan. It is tightly encased with fascia (connective tissue), dense, and it firmly adheres to the underlying muscle or bone as well as the overlying skin.

In contrast, the yellow fat I see is vivid in color, blobby and shapeless, and greasy to the touch.

Yellow fat is crummy-quality fat. Brown fat is good-quality fat. And the quality of your fat cannot be overestimated. The better your fat, the better you look and feel.

Having spent so many years working with subcutaneous brown fat to recontour the body, I instantly realized that this brown fat has several similar characteristics to the brown fat found deeper in the body as described in the recent studies. Namely, that lean people (with a lower body mass index, or BMI) have more brown fat than yellow fat, and that brown fat is directly related to control of your blood sugar.

While my goals and the goals of these scientists are the same—to use our own body's fat to reshape and revitalize—our methods of harnessing brown fat's power are different. The brown-fat researchers look forward to developing a drug to control this functionally active brown fat, which would be an incredible breakthrough for the health of millions of overweight people. But because their studies are still so new, these researchers have understandably admitted that developing any sort of drug to trigger deep brown fat's thermogenic properties is still years away—and that it might actually be impossible to create one.

The happy news is that the Brown Fat Revolution is available right now, and it works. I have spent years developing this program to help you replace your old, unhealthy yellow fat with new, healthy brown fat that is the hallmark of youthful volume.

WHY BROWN FAT IS EVEN MORE IMPORTANT AS YOU GROW OLDER

The *quality* of your body fat changes naturally with age, from young, light brown fat to old yellow fat. For women going through perimenopause and beyond, when the hormonally triggered changes they experience can be as bewildering and debilitating as puberty once was, the volume distribution or placement of their body fat will change as they age, too. This is the reason why so many of my patients over the age of forty have pointed to their bellies, telling me that they've grown a pooch seemingly overnight, and then begged me, as Lisa did, to help them.

Often, before they've come to see me, these patients have tried just about everything. First they panic. Then they start starving themselves. Then they work themselves into a frenzy in the gym.

But what happens? They feel awful and look worse. Their skin loses its luster, so their faces look gaunt and pinched. Instead of getting more energy from exercise, they're exhausted and crabby all the time. They've overexercised so much that, believe it or not, their faces are literally paying the price. Although they had good intentions and the discipline to make a strong commitment to health, they unwittingly chose the wrong strategy toward their fat, so it became impossible for them to achieve their goals.

All because they thought fat was the enemy.

When your body has the right proportions of good brown fat, you will always look youthful. The flip side, of course, is that if your body has the wrong proportions of bad yellow fat, you will always look soft, flabby, and old before your time.

Understanding the difference between brown and yellow fat is the heart of this book, because how you look as you age is *not* based on your weight. Thin does not always translate to looking young, because shape and contour define youth. Instead, your youthfulness is based on your proportions, and how your hormones determine where brown and yellow fat shifts in your body as you grow older.

In other words, when you follow the plans in *The Brown Fat Revolution*, you'll realize that what they target is your *shape*. You'll not only lose weight, but you'll regain the shapeliness that is the hallmark of youth.

When your shape is firm, lifted, and curvy, supported by the good brown fat you're soon going to have, you will always look younger. Once you start following the unique Eating and Exercise Plans in this book, you will never need a surgeon to get rid of your unhealthy yellow fat the way Lisa needed me.

The principles you'll read about will help you maintain the best balance of fat and muscle, and keep as high a proportion of brown fat to yellow fat as possible in order to hold on to the curves of femininity and the firmness and lift of youth, no matter what your age. And because this good brown fat will firmly support your skin, making it more youthful throughout your body, you'll also see the following:

- Your face will show improved tone and contour.

- Your arms will look more toned due to the loss of yellow fat and the formation of well-toned, firm muscles. Your belly will flatten due to decreased internal yellow fat.

- Your upper back will be smoother, and the area where your arms join your back will no longer be puffing over the sides of your bra.

- If you have cellulite, it will definitely show a marked improvement once the skin there is supported with healthy, firm young fat, and not mushy, old yellow fat.

- You will literally de-age yourself, solely by the way you eat and exercise. Not only will you improve your health, you'll enhance your beauty at the same time.

WHY THIS BOOK IS UNIQUE

Most anti-age books talk about the need for exercise and good skin care. But they concentrate on either the health benefits of exercise (such as using it along with diet to help you try to lose weight), or on the beautifying aspects of your appearance (with, for example, a certain kind of skin-care regimen). Many exercise books are written by certified trainers who concentrate only on movement and some kind of diet, without understanding the entire picture of physiology and metabolism—and certainly not the difference between yellow and brown fat. Many nutritionists write books because they want to help you lose weight, but although they understand metabolic functions, they don't usually understand the crucial role of yellow and brown fat, either. Even more important, many nutritionists do not design programs to specifically shape the body in addition to helping you lose weight. They design programs so that you'll lose fat and overall weight.

The reason for this is that most medical professionals don't think of fat the same way I do, as wanting to understand fat and the language of volume has shaped my entire career. I first became interested in the body's fat when I studied anatomy in medical school, and my interest progressed during my three decades of experience in shaping bodies with a scalpel and my two hands.

I'm assuming that anybody who reads my book wants to lose weight. But that's not enough for me—I want you to lose weight *and* look more youthful and more vibrant at the same time. Believe me, it can be done. Making tremendous, noticeable changes to your health and to your appearance is no longer an either/or situation.

Unlike most of my colleagues, I know what you need to do to not only feel better and lose weight—but also look incredible. The better you look, the better you're going to feel, which will keep you on the program until it's second nature.

My goal with this book is to have you completely rethink your attitude toward fat, and understand that young, healthy brown fat is a good thing.

HOW THIS BOOK WORKS

The Brown Fat Revolution will give you a concise explanation of the external and internal changes to your fat (and the rest of your body) as you age, coupled with a no-fail plan showing you how to use this knowledge to combat aging. You'll learn that what you eat has a direct effect on the *quality* of your fat, and how you exercise has a direct effect on the *quantity* of your fat. You'll get rid of bad yellow fat not by dieting or starving or spending endless, fruitless hours in the gym, but by alternating Protein Days with Carbohydrate Days, and increasing your metabolism with lean muscle.

Because hormones have the most profound effect on how our bodies age, each part of this book contains sections on two categories: Hormone Category I (ages thirty to fifty) and Hormone Category II (fifty and older). Chapters 2 and 3 will go into greater detail about hormones and the aging process. Armed with this information, you can then turn to the section of the book that is most applicable to your unique needs, and for quicker results you can target the areas of your body where the bad yellow fat has accumulated.

In part 1 you get the primer on fat, based on my thirty years of clinical experience studying the human body, as well as details of how your body ages.

Part 2 explains how the Eating Plan works, and why eating fat is good for you—as long as it's the right kind of fat. Once you start following this plan, you'll actually be eating a lot more while weighing less. Optimal nourishment will give you skin that glows, and a face that retains its youthful curves instead of looking haggard and aged.

Part 3 is all about replacing bad yellow fat with good brown fat through a revolutionary, time-efficient Exercise Plan that proves you can become fit and strong without spending hours each day on exercise.

Combining the Eating Plan with the Exercise Plan will provide maximum benefits. You won't be hungry, plus you'll raise your metabolism to a steady level so you won't gain weight. You'll no longer build up deposits of bad yellow fat, so you will quickly see results as a healthy underpinning of dense brown fat helps improve skin tone, decrease wrinkles, and minimize cellulite. Once you learn how to sculpt and strengthen your body without punishing your face, you'll be able to maintain this healthy, glowing, toned, firm skin without needing expensive procedures.

THE BROWN FAT REVOLUTION IS A PLAN FOR LIFE

Let me tell you another story about fat. My *own* fat.

I had been a competitive ballroom dancer as a teenager, eventually becoming the National Junior Latin and International Champion, but once I got into medical school, I stopped dancing. For the next twenty-two years, as I finished my medical training and opened my practice, I did nothing physical.

Nor did I pay close attention to what I put in my mouth, or how much. On a typical day, I'd finish my hours of grueling surgery and I'd be *hungry*. I'd go into the hospital lounge, looking for the usual plate of cookies and other treats. But I wouldn't eat just a cookie or two to take the edge off my hunger—I'd eat half a box while waiting for my nurse, Dede, to get me a steak sandwich and a few Hostess Sno Balls that I'd hide from my colleagues.

Or I'd hit the Mallomars. I was so addicted to them that if you'd told me back then that I'd lose my craving, I'd have looked at you as if you'd grown another head!

I was still fairly thin, but I was developing a Pillsbury Doughboy belly. I didn't feel great, either. My temper was short. I yelled at my staff for the most innocuous reasons. Something had to give.

That's when, at age forty, I started to work out. I found a gym some distance away so no one I knew would see me. My first day, one of the trainers—a gymnast named Rick—came in, and I asked him to work with me.

But I still wasn't really concentrating, because the only time I could schedule our sessions was in the early morning, which is when I did my surgeries, and I felt so guilty because I wasn't working.

Finally, Rick got fed up. "What the hell's up with you?" he asked. "If you can't devote one hour two or three lousy times a week to yourself, you have a *pathetic* life."

I laughed to cover up my mortification, because I knew he was right. But it still took a few more months before I truly began to change my thinking. I was done with quick fixes and quack diets. I was on a mission—to develop a program that would keep me fit, make me healthy again, and have the astonishing side benefit of completely changing the way I looked. A program that would work, that would continue to improve my health and appearance—for life.

I was also determined to make the Brown Fat Revolution foolproof. With this program no longer will you feel a sense of depravation and obligation—you'll feel empowered and positive once you see how easy it is to reverse the effects of bad yellow fat and start replacing it with good brown fat. Because the steps are clearly listed, you won't have to think about what to eat or how to exercise. If you stick to the program, you *cannot* fail.

Good brown fat is transformative. With it, you'll be able to rebuild, replenish, restore, and recontour your body, put the bloom back on your skin, and add vitality back to your life.

My mission is not just to diminish your overall fat volume, but to help you replace it with a healthy and attractive volume of high-quality fat, a fat that looks brown due to its inherent architecture. A fat that is akin to the brown fat that is presently under scientific investigation as a means of controlling weight. This is a very promising role for those fat cells once thought to be the enemy of obesity!

PART I

THE BROWN FAT REVOLUTION BASICS

1.
THE SCIENCE BEHIND THE BROWN FAT REVOLUTION

Fat is your friend.

I'm determined to help you rethink what your fat is. It might take some time to wrap your mind around that idea, but the simple truth is that everyone needs fat. Not a diet that's fat-free. Not a diet that's low-fat. Not a diet fueled by the notion of "I'll get fat if I eat fat."

You need good, nutritious, healthful fats in your food. And you need good, firm, resilient brown fat in your body—not the old yellow fat that's basically mush—for not just optimum health but optimum beauty, too. The difference between young fat and old fat is like the difference between a smooth round plum and a wrinkled prune. One is dense, smooth, and rounded, and the other is not.

Furthermore, the recently published studies on deep, functional brown fat provide clear evidence that, ironically, the answer to the obesity epidemic may be more straightforward than formerly thought. For these scientists, the answer lies in the fat cell itself!

So let's take a look at the crucial role of fat—and what you can do about getting rid of old yellow fat and replacing it with new brown fat.

WE'RE OBSESSED WITH FAT—BUT FOR ALL THE WRONG REASONS

Too many people in our country are becoming alarmingly obese. Cookbooks and health books and talk shows and magazine articles are constantly bombarding us with images and facts about the fat that causes diseases—and kills. There is, in fact, a particular mindset where it's all too easy to see fat as the enemy without understanding how and why the right kind of fat is so important. And because many people do not understand what nutrients the body needs and when to eat them, they end up eating all the wrong things, and put on more weight. Or they become alarmingly thin, somehow thinking that starving themselves of all fat is the only way to achieve that superflat belly and those jutting cheekbones.

But the *right* fat in the right areas is a good thing. It's an intrinsic part of your body. If you want to feel good and look good, it's essential to have a body where all systems are functioning at optimum levels, both physically and mentally.

Just as important: understanding that eating the right kind of fat will not make you fatter.

That is, you will not get fatter if you eat the kind of fat that's good for your body; eat it at the right times during the day, along with carbohydrates, to keep your metabolism on an even keel; and don't eat so much of it that your body automatically stores it instead of burning it off.

So when did we make the switch from looking at adorable little babies with rolls of fat on their thighs, wanting to blow on their dumpling bellies to make them peal with laughter . . . to being afraid to eat properly and obsessing about every calorie we put in our mouths, even as we struggle to maintain a healthy weight or a figure with curves where we want them?

I've spent many hours trying to figure out when fat became a four-letter word. I clearly remember the day when the daughter of a family friend was over, and my wife and I were watching a Marilyn Monroe movie. This teenager had never seen Marilyn in her prime before. And

MICHELLE OBAMA HAS GREAT FAT; MADONNA DOESN'T

Michelle Obama has an amazing body—not because it's got the most amazing shape, but because she's amazingly average, with exactly the right amount of good brown fat in her face and body.

It's interesting to take a look at her figure, as she's got broad shoulders, a small bust, and a small waist, yet wide hips, an ample butt, and long legs. She's not skinny, and she's not fat—she's firm and toned, with exceptionally well-defined upper arms. She exudes health and vitality. Her posture is perfect and she carries herself with elegance and grace. Most of all, she's a woman comfortable in her own skin.

Compare Michelle's lovely strong curves with Madonna's angular, supermuscled and almost terrifyingly buff body. Although Madonna is only five years Michelle's senior, she looks much older, because she has almost no body fat at all. Unless she's carefully lit in photographs, she can look harsh, haggard, and tired.

In other words, Michelle Obama has got great fat. Madonna doesn't. That doesn't mean I don't admire Madonna for her singing and dancing talent, her staggering discipline, her work ethic, and her seemingly inexhaustible energy and stamina. Personally, I believe that if Madonna stopped her compulsively long workouts (a reported minimum of four hours a day) and gained about fifteen pounds, she would look so spectacular she'd knock your socks off.

what was the girl's response? That Marilyn was sexy, or beautiful, or vulnerable? I wish! Instead, she said, "Oh my God. She's so *fat*!"

It was a disheartening moment, I have to say, as Marilyn's glorious curves are certainly not what I'd consider to be "fat." And, as someone who's devoted his life to optimum health, it pains me to look at images of seriously underweight and undernourished Hollywood stars, with their toothpick legs, pin-thin arms, and cheeks that are rounded due not to good brown fat but to the miracles of modern medicine, which has created the kind of substances that can be injected or inserted into them to plump them up. I'm left wondering how these stars can continue to function with such patently unhealthy bodies—and what kind of role models they are for the women of the world.

Frankly, I think thin is bad. You can't be a stick and be healthy. And the older you get, the more aging this gaunt thinness becomes.

I have an intimate knowledge of the danger of thinness, because as a plastic surgeon, I deal with it on a daily basis. From my point of view, what I do for a living is plump up thin faces, and put implants in areas of the body perceived by their owners to be too thin, whether their cheeks or their jaws, their breasts or their butts. Not that any of this is wrong, of course. But what, really, is the heart of the issue?

It's fat, of course!

FAT BASICS

Your body intrinsically knows, within the modulation of its metabolism, how much fat it needs to function. Anything beyond that will be stored for future use, to supply energy when needed.

Your body prefers to store energy as fat, as a direct result of tens of thousands of years of evolution. Early humans had trouble finding food, especially calorie-dense food. Plus they were in constant motion as they went hunting every day. As fat is calorie dense, with nine kilocalories per gram (carbohydrates and protein each have four kilocalories per gram), it became the most efficient way to provide the stored energy our ancestors needed for survival.

Fast-forward to the present, when we're no longer hunter/gatherers and have every conceivable food at our fingertips. While we've evolved enough to create art and music and send a man to the moon, the human body's technology has not evolved at the same pace. It still thinks it's going to have to hunt for its next meal, so it will always hoard all excess calories in the form of fat—if you let it.

WHY YOU NEED FAT

Fat is necessary for several basic bodily functions. Your body needs a certain amount of fat to store the vitamins A, D, E, and K, which are necessary to maintain the health of your cell membranes and its walls, as well as the overall health of skin, bones, and the immune and clotting systems. Bodies must also have fat for the brain and the neuro-system, so nerves can fire properly and communicate with each other. This is why it's so important for babies to have a lot of fat in their diets; without it, their brains won't develop properly.

With only a minimal amount of fat in your body, you won't feel very well and you'll look horrible. Your skin will be dull, your immune system will be compromised, and your energy level will be nonexistent.

I've seen the horrifying effects of a superstrict no-fat diet in the bodybuilders who train at my gym. In the weeks before a competition, these guys starve themselves to make their muscles look more ripped. Not only is this unhealthy, but their faces become so drawn and pale, it's not an exaggeration to say that they look like they're dying. Their brains are so starved for fat and carbohydrates that their synapses aren't firing properly. They tell me they feel like they're out of control. Basically, they are, as they literally can't think straight.

ABOUT INSULIN, GLYCOGEN,
AND WHAT CAUSES YELLOW FAT

Since your body will always store excess calories as fat, if you eat too much of any food that is converted into fat, it's converted into the kind of bad yellow fat you don't want.

Think of your food as coal being added to a furnace. If you add too much coal, the fire gets too hot and then burns out. If there's always way too much coal, the bottom of the pile will become powdered and useless, similar to low-quality yellow fat.

Whenever you eat carbohydrates, your body secretes insulin, the hormone that regulates blood sugar, to maintain an even blood-sugar level. Insulin wants excess sugars out of the blood, so it immediately spikes and then falls to move the excess someplace less harmful—like your fat cells. Your *yellow* fat cells.

An additional part of the process has to do with glycogen, the name for your body's initial stores of carbohydrates. Most glycogen is stored in the liver and muscles, and released when your body needs it. In other words, glycogen is an energy source that is immediately available so your brain can function well and your muscles can move where you want them to.

If you eat the right amount of food, your body will not need to store any excess calories, which are always stored as fat. Instead, it will store the calories only as glycogen. When glycogen storage is exceeded, the extra glucose is deposited as fat. At first, it's deposited into good, brown fat cells. Healthy brown fat tissue is well contained in a framework of fascia, which keeps fat in a tight cluster supporting the overlying skin and firmly attached to the underlying muscles. There is a defined level at which fat tissue can maintain a homeostatic relationship with the surrounding fascia, blood supply, and lymphatic drainage—the three work together to create the shapes of youth in the face and body.

Now, fat cells do not increase in number as we gain weight. They only get larger. If you overeat, eat poorly, or don't exercise, excess fat increases in volume. As the fascia stretches, the fat starts to fall off the muscles and does not buttress the skin with the same firmness. If the cells become too enlarged, the fascia stretches along with the connective tissue holding the cells together and thinning of the nutrient blood vessels cannot contain the cell volume and the shape and tone, so they start to look loose and yellow—shapeless. The scale of fat quality is a continuum, from brown to yellow. Yellow fat *is* brown fat turned bad.

So if you eat too much, your insulin will keep on desperately trying to get the excess sugars out of your blood, and you'll never be able to deplete your glycogen stores to trigger the conversion process from bad yellow fat to good brown fat. Instead, you'll just get fatter and fatter in an endless cycle of blood-sugar highs and lows followed by increased storage of yellow fat.

As you'll learn in chapter 4, figuring out the balance of glycogen storage (to prevent excess consumed calories being stored as fat) with glycogen availability (to give you energy and to avoid any breakdown of your muscles) will be the foundation of your Eating Plan. Mobilizing glycogen for energy use is determined more by diet than by exercise.

The evolutionary "excess calories automatically get stored as fat" phenomenon is the basis of understanding yo-yo dieting. If you stick to a very calorie- and fat-restrictive diet, your body will automatically click into starvation mode, lessening its daily caloric need. Yet even when you start to eat normally again, your body will remain less efficient at processing the nutrients, and you'll quickly gain weight, and then some. Then you go back to a superrestrictive diet to lose the weight, and the vicious cycle of yo-yo dieting spirals out of control.

In addition, those who work out like crazy but don't eat properly will shrink in an unhealthy fashion; since they rapidly deplete their glycogen, they end up burning both fat and muscle for energy. Their bodies read the lack of glycogen as starvation, so their metabolism slows down, too. And those who work out like crazy but eat too much do not lose weight because as their glycogen is replenished, their appetites increase. As soon as they replenish their glycogen stores, any excess calories turn into yellow fat.

Your body weight is not the only indicator that you may have a lot of bad yellow fat. Sometimes those who are only very slightly overweight, who appear to be in excellent health, who have normal blood work and blood pressure and no inclination toward type 2 diabetes, have too-high yellow fat stores. Yet the damage that's going on hasn't been noticed yet because it's all *internal*. It's like a car that stalls suddenly for no apparent reason, and you've got no idea the engine is about to blow up!

CONVERTING YELLOW FAT TO BROWN FAT

Since you know that once your glycogen stores are all filled up, any other calories that come into the body are going to automatically be stored as yellow fat, the trick is to keep this glycogen storage level as close to even as possible. Have too little fat and carbohydrates, and you'll go into starvation mode. Have too much and you'll develop too much yellow fat.

What you want instead is healthy brown fat.

When you add fuel slowly and continuously, the fire in your body's furnace will burn evenly and steadily. Our bodies are designed to burn fat preferentially, so if the bad yellow fat becomes the most available form of fuel—in other words, when you can use it up instead of storing it—it will keep on getting burned up. Instead of losing muscle, healthy brown fat, and bone, as happens on most restrictive diets, all you'll lose is your bad yellow fat.

At the same time, when you eat nutritionally sound foods like complex carbohydrates, your body's need for the fat it must have for cell functions remains stable. With a constant and even concentration of glycogen in the muscles and liver, the body now thinks that glucose is no longer needed, so it's not immediately stored as bad yellow fat.

Our bodies "make" brown fat the same way we make all our tissues healthy anywhere. So instead of just thinking about *losing* pounds as you would during a typical weight-loss diet, I want you to be thinking about fat *replacement*, too—as in replacing yellow fat with dense brown fat.

That's because, as you know, the right volume in the right place is what makes you look shapely and youthful. Brown fat is not about weight—it's about *shape*.

WHAT DO YELLOW FAT AND BROWN FAT LOOK LIKE?

From my perspective as a surgeon with thirty years of experience cutting into bodies of all shapes and sizes, it's immediately apparent that yellow fat and brown fat look and feel and behave very differently.

If you look at yellow fat under a microscope, it's all white. It appears to have large vacuoles, which are large spaces inside a cell. The cell walls are stretched and there's very little fibrous tissue or blood vessels.

When I cut through yellow fat during surgery, there's little to no bleeding, which is very unhealthy; it's an indicator of how bad eating habits have a visible effect on the health of your tissues, even when you can't see them on the surface. Seeing yellow fat on the inside is like seeing the leathery, wrinkled skin on the outside of a woman who smokes and tans too much.

When I'm performing surgery on a healthy female patient, however—one who's nourished herself well and exercised often—I don't see yellow fat. I see firm brown fat in certain areas of the body—the areas that define the patient's gender.

Your body has well-defined areas where fat cells are located: on top of the muscles (subcutaneous, deep fat), in the abdomen (intra-abdominal fat), and in the organs (like the fat in the liver, for example). We're born with the number of fat cells, or adipocytes, that we'll carry through life; these cells can get larger or smaller as you gain or lose weight, but they can't multiply.

In each area, there is a predetermined network of connective tissue to organize and form the fat cells, a certain number of blood vessels to supply the fat with nutrients, and a certain number of lymphatics to drain the fatty tissue. If the size of the fat cells does not overwhelm the network of connective tissue; if the blood supply keeps up with the metabolism of each cell so it functions at the optimal metabolic rate; and if the size of the cells does not overwhelm the lymphatic drainage channels, you have brown fat.

Brown fat gets its color from thick, fibrous tissue between its cells, as well as countless blood vessels. As a result, it looks brown—more of a tan color, actually—because blood is constantly supplying and replenishing the fibrous tissue and fat.

In addition, brown fat is compact and shapely. It *looks* youthful (because it is). Brown fat adheres tightly to the overlying skin and underlying muscles. This cohesive relationship of skin, fat, and muscle defines youth!

With yellow fat, on the other hand, the network of connective tissue is overstretched due to the enormous fat cells, the equally stretched blood vessels course scantily through the cells, and cell membranes are loose and sometimes fragmented due to sluggish cellular metabolism that gets little nourishment because there's no blood to supply it. Yellow fat actually feels greasy as a result. Nor does it support the overlying skin or have the resilience to help contour the underlying muscles. It's blobby, with no defined volume. Or rather, its volume translates to old!

You can easily get an idea of what old yellow fat looks like every time you see a raw steak. When raw, the thick lumps of fat on the end are a dense, opaque white. It's got a very specific kind of greasy feel to it when you touch it.

On a raw chicken, yellow fat is definitely bright yellow, and in big clumps that you can pull out of the cavity or trim near the tail. Many chickens, though, don't have a lot of visible yellow fat anymore, as they've been bred to be extra-lean. Which is a good thing for you.

(Moral of the story: Always trim your meat. The kind of fat that's bad for you looks pretty gross on the outside—and you don't want it on your insides!)

YELLOW FAT IS PERVASIVE, TOO

One of the biggest problems with yellow fat is that it's pervasive. It moves into your vital organs, and particularly into your abdomen area and around your intestines. This pervasiveness is basically why people who are overweight have so many health problems. The quality of their tissues is poor; their metabolism is sluggish; and there's an increased demand on the heart and lungs. The body is in chronic overload, as if it's a truck dragging an entire house behind it all the time.

I was reminded of the pervasiveness of yellow fat when I was discussing it with a patient recently, and she told me about an incident that happened to her decades before, when she had gone to the hospital for some severe endocrine problems and had shared a room with several other patients, including a morbidly obese woman. This woman urgently needed a liver biopsy, normally a simple procedure done under local anesthesia, so one day the surgeon and his team came into the room, drew the curtains around her bed, and sedated her. They got to work, and then a few minutes later there was an ungodly crash. The surgeon came stomping out, his face beet red, swearing at the top of his lungs. What had happened? He'd been unable to find this woman's liver. Her yellow fat had completely obscured her internal organs.

Anyway, this hot-tempered surgeon got so frustrated—inappropriately so, I might add—that he knocked the instruments to the floor. But I could understand his frustration, because he wanted the best for this woman. He knew her life was now at grave risk because she'd have to have general anesthesia for a simple biopsy.

The bottom line is, there is never going to be any need for yellow fat. We don't need it to give us energy—we have glycogen and good brown fat for that. So beyond what you look like, it increases your need for insulin, makes you prone to diabetes, makes you feel sluggish, and may increase your risk during medical procedures. It is intermingled with all tissues of your body—your heart, liver, everywhere. It's pretty gross.

THE SKINNY ON FAT

Anyone who's seen a recent fashion show knows that the runway models are so skinny you could seemingly blow them over like a feather—but they've also got jiggly bottoms and wobbly thighs. Why? Because they don't eat enough, or they don't eat properly when they do eat, and many don't exercise. (Believe me, I'm not blaming them—I'm blaming the fashion industry.) So the tiny amount of fat these models have is mushy yellow fat. These women are barely out of their teens, a size 00, yet they're fat and skinny at the same time.

Superskinny models are the visible embodiment of yellow fat versus brown fat. That they deprive themselves of good nutrition means they don't have good-quality tissue. Just as skin will reflect damage done to it by smoking and excessive tanning and look old before its time, doing the wrong things to the tissues of your body will be visible, too. Poor-quality tissues, such as yellow fat, are going to look and act a certain way whether there's too much of them (as in an overweight person) or too little (as in a severely underweight person).

Next time there's a Hollywood award show on TV, watch the actresses walking down the red carpet—you know, the actresses who are lovely, gorgeous, talented, and starving. See who's very thin, yet still has a little pooch in the front. That's bad yellow fat.

Even though these actresses often follow vigorous exercise regimens, they don't know how to target the excess yellow fat in their abdomens or butts and replace it with healthy brown fat. Their bodies are desperate for any fat at all—so they'll hold on to whatever they can get. This is due to a condition called lipodystrophy, the hormone-driven phenomenon responsible for areas of collected fat in certain areas of the body. These areas are the most resistant areas to weight loss, and need a little push—namely the Brown Fat Revolution program.

Yellow fat has no purpose except to, well, hang there and make you feel miserable and look older.

TOO LITTLE FAT

While I can't do much about the bodybuilders who are starving themselves before a competition, I can try to do something about the countless patients who erroneously think that avoiding fat or severely restricting calories will help them get or remain superthin.

If you don't have enough of the good brown fat, you'll get way too thin—not attractively lean, but scary skinny!

Without fat for energy, you'll have minimal glycogen stores in your body. Then if you decide to work out, you'll deplete all your stored glycogen, and your muscles won't work properly. They'll be too weak. And weak muscles can't get stronger, so you won't put on any of the lean muscle mass that makes you look youthful and strong.

But the Brown Fat Revolution is designed to replenish these glycogen stores throughout the day, to keep the fuel burning evenly. Which is why it's absolutely essential to eat a postworkout meal, as this will supply instant calories for your muscles so they'll be able not only to replenish themselves, but to prevent the stressed muscles from cannibalizing other muscles after the demands of the workout.

With the Eating Plan, you'll keep your metabolism evenly burning and therefore working most efficiently, so your body won't be converting calories into fat deposits. It won't need to. And that's when the weight will finally come off—and stay off.

FAT: IT'S ALL ABOUT THE VOLUME

My son Blake used to be on his college dive team, so he gets what makes muscles work and become shapely with the right kind of weight training; and after listening to me discuss my theories over the years, he gets metabolism and brown and yellow fat.

"Fat is the language of volume," he told me. "Because volume is created by fat."

And volume is what makes us look youthful.

If you close your eyes and envision a twenty-year-old face and a fifty-five-year-old face, then erase all the wrinkles from their skin, which face will appear older?

The twenty-year-old face will be round and curvy. The fifty-five-year-old face will be thinner and more angular. It'll look older due not to the amount of wrinkles, but to its shape, lost volume, and the distribution of fat.

Having the right amount of good brown fat that will keep you looking and feeling youthful is like building a house with a strong and sturdy foundation. You want a structurally sound house—and you want a structurally sound body, too. If you don't create a solid structure that will properly support what's built upon it, anything you do to the surface will be cosmetic only. It's like painting a house without priming it first—the paint will soon peel and flake, leaving the raw wood exposed to the elements and ruining your house.

FAT AND YOUR FACE

You need good brown fat supporting the tissues in your face to create a soft, youthful look. Losing this fat as you grow older changes the volume of your face, making it look gaunt. Despite what cosmetics companies often claim, their moisturizers and creams can treat only the outer layers of your skin—they can't treat the underlying tissues, so there's nothing you can buy over the counter to replace lost volume in your face.

THE FAT AND FAT POCKETS OF YOUR FACE

What surgeons have learned is that you don't have one solid sheet of fat under your skin, although it looks like that when you're young. Instead, there are several fat "pockets" that all have their own internal aging clock. The different pockets of fat gain and lose volume separately, and sag with gravity at different rates—explaining why your face doesn't age uniformly.

Although you have no control over how these pockets of fat in your face are going to age, since you can't control the pull of gravity, you *do* have the ultimate control over how you affect them—by the way you behave. And the way *not* to behave is by losing all your good brown fat. As you know, brown fat creates volume and plumps up skin to make you look youthful. So when you get rid of bad yellow fat and replace it with dense brown fat, it will make a startling improvement to the shape of your face.

AGING FROM THE TOP DOWN

Let's divide the face into four segments, so you can more clearly understand how it ages: the forehead, the eye area, the cheeks, and the central face (the lips and chin, or perioral area, meaning around the mouth).

These four segments are all unique, especially in texture; the forehead skin is fairly thick, while eyelid skin is more like silk, and cheek skin is smooth and peachy. They age at different rates, because they're affected by different processes. Foreheads and the perioral skin, for example, respond to the constant movements of the muscles underneath; eyelids are affected by wrinkling and by fat; cheeks are affected by how the fat gradually slides down toward the jawline.

The key point is that the four segments usually age *from the top down*. This is relevant to understanding fat because what fills your face with volume, what supports your skin and creates the undulations of youth, is brown fat. With age, facial fat descends, diminishes in quality, and becomes more yellow in consistency.

Improve the quality of your facial fat, and your face will automatically look better. Dense, toned brown fat hugs the bones and muscles and intimately supports the overlying skin; lose the coalescence of these tissues and you'll have a face that truly shows its age.

Aging from the top down happens externally and internally, on the topical level of your skin itself and to the underlying structure of fat, muscle, and bone. Most often, you'll first see wrinkles on the forehead, then on the eyelids, then in the crow's-feet area, then the cheeks, and then the nasolabial fold, or the line running from your nose down to your lips.

As we get older, vertical lines—what I call the elevens—start to appear between your brows and in the deepening of the nasolabial folds. You'll also see the eyebrows descending, the cheeks losing shapeliness, and the chin line becoming less defined and more jowly.

To me, the cheeks are the most interesting part of the aging face, as well as the most difficult part to correct without the correction being obvious. That's because the volume of the cheek, the beautiful curve right over the cheekbone in the apple (referred to in medical terminology as an ogee curve), which then descends down to the mouth segment, has nothing to do with skin. It has everything to do with *fat*.

I like to call the aging of the cheek "devolution." The fat actually flattens out and falls down, leaving a hollowing-out under the eye. The apple descends and creates a jowl, as if it were dripping fat like wax melting down a candle.

Restoring the quantity and quality of the volume in your cheeks is what truly creates a youthful contour, whether you're thirty or seventy.

FAT AND YOUR BODY

Aging from the top down doesn't just affect your face. Your entire body starts to, well, droop from the neck down to your torso and eventually reaching your ankles and feet—primarily due, of course, to changes in fat distribution. But, as you've figured out by now, only if you let it!

The controlling factor when it comes to the distribution of fat in the aging process is your hormones. They're responsible for the shape of your body, whether it's 99, 150, or 250 pounds.

ABOUT HORMONES

Estrogen is the female hormone that rules all other female hormones, particularly during its profound fluctuations during puberty, pregnancy, and perimenopause/menopause.

The amount of estrogen your body produces will define your fat distribution. It's that simple—and the reason why men and women put on weight differently.

When a young girl moves toward puberty and gets her first period, she'll start to deposit fat in her thighs. During the ensuing decades of fertility, fat will obviously be distributed in the breasts and abdomen during pregnancy. As estrogen as well as progesterone levels begin to decline, changes in fat distribution become even more pronounced. At the same time, the male hormones, or androgens (which all women have), become more pronounced, triggering the movement of fat to areas like the arms, the front of the neck, the sides of the breasts, and the central abdomen.

Obviously, hormonal changes are happening slowly over time, and there's no predicting how you'll fare during your lifetime. But it must be said that if your health isn't good, if you don't eat well, and if you don't exercise, chances are much higher that you'll suffer more extreme symptoms as menopause approaches, because you'll have less brown fat and more of the yellow fat that wreaks havoc on your body.

THE REST OF THE BODY AGES, TOO

Why do we age?

Basically, all of the structures of our bodies are held together in a toned fashion by elastic fibers and collagen. Together, they make up the "scaffolding" of what we call connective tissue. The matrix, or substance that surrounds the elastic fibers and collagen, is made up of mucopolysaccharides, which are what hold water in tissue. Think of it as the fabric or the netting in between cells. With age, the connective tissue loosens and becomes more lax.

While there's nothing you can do about the fact that collagen and elastin are going to degrade over time, you can certainly retard the process by living and eating well. A fifty-year-old woman who's in good shape and who's never smoked is much more likely to look vibrant and youthful than an overweight smoker, due to the better quality of her connective tissue. It's why such a woman will have a younger "Visual Age" than her overweight, smoking counterpart who is the same chronological age.

Ideally, you want to have a Visual Age that is lower than your chronological age. You'll certainly be able to do that when you follow the Eating and Exercise Plans in this book.

How your skeleton holds up over the years is one of the basic markers of aging. Bones tend to demineralize and therefore get softer over time, especially in women. This can be exacerbated if you're calcium deficient, leading to osteoporosis. If the osteoporosis is extreme, you literally lose inches of height.

Your organs also work less productively as you age. This has nothing to do with fat. Believe me, if scientists could figure out how to stave off these inexorable changes, we would all live a lot longer.

WHY "SPOT REDUCING" IS A FALLACY

There's no such thing as "spot reducing"—but I can't tell you how many of my patients think that if they do a lot of crunches, their bellies are going to get thinner. Or that if they do a lot of arm exercises, their arms will lose fat, too.

Your body is predisposed to put on fat in certain areas, and from a physiological point of view, there's just not anything you can do about it. But—and this is the crucial *but*—if you have good brown fat in the areas where fat tends to be visible (like the belly), you won't really notice it. It will lie flat near your muscles. It will be dense and resilient and supportive, so you won't get that droopiness or pooching that you associate with getting older. It will create the curves and shadows of a healthy, attractive body.

AND NOW . . . ONWARD TO THE BROWN FAT REVOLUTION

What is the essence of the Brown Fat Revolution?

When it comes to fat, what do we all want to do? We want to control the volume of fat in our bodies as well as the quality of this fat. We also want to have faces and bodies that are as healthy and youthful-looking as possible.

So why do people get fat? The principle is simple: You put on fat when you put more energy into your body (with food) than you put out (with energy expended, as with exercise). But the solution to managing fat in/fat out is not simple at all—which is why obesity is at epidemic levels. The average American doesn't know how to eat well or when, or how much exercise to do and what exercises will be best for them.

The Brown Fat Revolution will show you that instead of thinking of fat as the enemy, you can learn how to harness its power to reshape your body and improve your health.

The Eating Plan will teach you that when you eat specific kinds of foods (either carbohydrates or protein) at specific times during the day, you won't have any excess carbohydrates left in your body to be converted into yellow fat.

Eating six times a day will keep your blood sugar at an even level, so you will avoid the peaks and valleys of cravings that lead to bingeing. Your body will quickly come to realize that more nutritious food will always be coming every few hours, so it will no longer be primed to store any excess as yellow fat. Calories will automatically become good brown fat.

The Exercise Plan will help you strengthen and shore up the nonbulky muscles of your core—all the muscles that define a youthful silhouette. Lean muscle has high energy requirements, so even at rest it will keep your metabolism elevated. (It's as if you'll be creating a muscle furnace!) Combine the new, stronger, leaner muscles with the balanced approach to eating, and you will not only get rid of your yellow fat, but also strengthen the rest of your body as well as improve your posture.

This system will work even if you have declining hormone levels—the hormones that trigger more fat deposits as you age. As you get older, your body preferentially deposits fat in specific sites, most noticeably the abdomen, flanks, outer thighs, and upper arms. (*When* this happens is determined by your genes and your gender.) But once you replace these hormone-triggered, "middle-age" zones of yellow fat with dense and resilient brown fat, your body will once again look younger and more shapely.

Read on, and you'll see how the Brown Fat Revolution will work for you.

2.
HOW YOU AGE—AND HOW FAT PLAYS ITS ROLE: HORMONE CATEGORY I

Now that you understand the crucial role of fat, let's take a look at what's going on inside your body—at the shifting patterns of your fat distribution, and other changes you'll experience as you age.

Because the aging concerns of women in the child-bearing years are different from those of women twenty years their seniors, there are two distinct Eating Plans for the Hormone I and Hormone II categories, as you'll see in part 2.

Women in their thirties have faces that show their experience yet are still stunningly youthful; the genetic traits that predispose them to certain skin conditions, such as dark undereye circles, usually have not yet appeared. Or, at least, there's no reason for their faces *not* to be youthful (unless the women have been chain-smoking or baking in the sun every day). Although getting older is not often at the top of any thirtysomething's to-do-with-enthusiasm list, by tackling the aging process *now*, you'll not only replace yellow fat with firm brown fat, but look and feel younger for much, much longer.

I often explain this concept to my patients in their thirties, but a lot of them don't listen—not until I add that it's inappropriate to treat things that do not exist yet, such as injecting Botox into as-yet-to-appear wrinkles on their foreheads. And that how their faces look is directly related to their overall health and sense of well-being.

For instance, for patients in their thirties who eat crummy food, drink too much, smoke, and are hugely stressed out, all the injectables in the world will not make a difference. The analogy I use is: Imagine that you ignored the health of your teeth until you were in your thirties. What would the dentist do when you appeared in his office when you were thirty-three? A competent dentist would never cover up the rotten teeth with shiny veneers. Instead, a good dentist would teach you about good dental health.

All the rejuvenating treatments I offer my patients are ineffectual without healthy living. Typical of those patients is Miranda. She's thirty-six, has a good but high-pressure job at a large corporation, and is busy dating and comparing notes with her girlfriends. She spends her summer weekends at the beach in the Hamptons and many of her winter weekends skiing in Vermont, occasionally remembering to use sunscreen. She often eats out in restaurants, entertaining clients, and has a glass or two of wine during these evenings. She wants to keep her job, so she takes great care to keep her energy up and look her best. She also wants to maintain her edge and sexiness, as she would very much like to find Mr. Right.

But she's doing all the wrong things. She—like most of her colleagues, or friends who are stay-at-home moms—rushes to the gym several days a week, exercising with lots of cardio (such as a high-intensity spinning class) and an abs class. She skips breakfast every day, grabs lunch on the run (usually a nonfat yogurt), barely touches fruit or vegetables, but drinks bottled water and coffee all day long and scarfs down whatever vitamins her friends tell her they've read about. Because she often has to eat out for work, she rarely cooks for herself. In fact, she likes to joke that her oven is a great place to store her shoes, as she never uses it.

Miranda came to see me because she's concerned that her skin looks "tired and blah," as she put it, and because she's worried that the "elevens" between her eyebrows as well as her nasolabial folds are deepening, making her look angry and tense all the time.

Although Miranda doesn't know it yet, she's on the tip of the critical mass iceberg, with her face undergoing subtle changes, most of which are not yet visible. Which is why she was not happy when I told her that, yes, a few injections of Botox would temporarily erase the wrinkles on her forehead, and a few syringes of Juvéderm injected into her nasolabial fold would help plump up the area, but that they wouldn't do anything about the bad yellow fat that's starting to wreak havoc in her face.

And that, in fact, if I used Botox and fillers, I'd be treating only her symptoms—*not* the cause of her complaint.

It was time to coach Miranda into a complete lifestyle change, one that would restore her skin to optimal condition; rehydrate her facial tissues, including her facial fat; optimize the volume relationships of the tissues of her face; and help her understand that she needed to treat her face and body as one unit. I explained that she had the power to control the process entirely through a much more nutritious Eating Plan and a much shorter and easier Exercise Plan that would utterly transform her face and body, delay the aging process, and help her look the best she possibly could—for the rest of her life. And that if she followed the plan, she would no longer need Botox or fillers, because the positive changes she'd make would enhance her face well beyond a level that could be achieved with these treatments alone.

Making this a program for life means taking the time for (and getting the emotional satisfaction from) doing what you mean when you say "My body is hugely valuable to me. I am going to respect and nourish my body now to keep it alive and thriving for as long as I possibly can." It's a very different mindset than "You fix it and I'll forget about it."

In fact, if you follow these Eating and Exercise Plans from the time you're thirty, you, like Miranda, will be sparing yourself the need for injectable fillers to replace the lost volume in your face once you turn fifty. Women in their thirties respond incredibly quickly to this plan. As long as you stay on it, once your yellow fat is transformed to brown fat, it will remain as brown fat, keeping your face and body firm and resilient, with strong, toned muscles.

You will, in essence, have created your own anti-aging regimen by slowing down the aging process, all on your own. Of course, you can't make yourself have good brown fat that looks thirty forever, but you can certainly stave off the unwelcome aspects of aging for far longer than you dreamed possible.

You won't just look far younger than your chronological age—your internal organs and your skin will *be* younger because, buoyed by their cushion of dense brown fat, you'll be in optimal health.

HOW YOU AGE IN YOUR THIRTIES AND FORTIES

"Critical mass" is a term used to describe a tipping point for your body, and it starts in your thirties. You will be undergoing very slow, incremental changes, particularly with the yellow fat deep inside your body, but they likely aren't yet noticeable, since your eye needs to see a certain amount of critical mass to visually connect to it. Without these visual cues, it's hard to believe these changes are truly happening.

You'll have experienced the critical-mass phenomenon every time old friends reconnect with you, either in person or on a social networking site like Facebook. The longer the time span between the last time you saw them and the present, the more pronounced your reaction will be to their current appearance. It can be jaw-droppingly scary to see old friends who appear to be aged well beyond their years, especially if they're the same age you are—and if your memories of them are of when they still had their youthful contours and strong, firm bodies. If, however, you'd seen these people every week for the last twenty years, you would be far less surprised at how they're aging.

Critical mass is also one of the reasons why it's so hard to convince women to wear sunscreen religiously. Unless they get a bad burn, they don't see the skin damage from the sun every day. It takes many years for spots, freckles, blotches, and wrinkles to develop. By the time they do appear, the real damage has been done—and undoing it is a lot more difficult than preventing the damage from happening in the first place.

So when you think about aging in your thirties and forties, remember that you might not yet be seeing the visible effects of aging—but they're lurking just beneath the surface, ready to appear, if you don't take action now.

CHANGES TO YOUR CELLS

Believe it or not, as soon as you're born, you start to die.

Your body is made up of trillions of cells, all with a set lifespan. How long they're able to function is called cell senescence, the biological equivalent of old age. In a young cell, its metabolism is active and the waste products produced are easily removed. In an old cell, its metabolism slows down and its ability to remove waste also decreases, so this waste can back up into the cell itself, leading to sluggishness. The cellular rate of reproduction decreases, and cell membranes are prone to breaking down more easily as well.

Due to critical mass, cell senescence doesn't create a visual change until it reaches a certain threshold. At that point, all these changes at the primal, cellular level have affected all your tissues, so you look different—and older.

The Brown Fat Revolution is designed to enhance cell metabolism, restore some of the essential cell functions, and therefore be able to reverse some of these visual changes. Lucky you if you're in your thirties—this program can delay the changes significantly, too.

CHANGES TO YOUR FAT

During your thirties, your fat should still be firm, unless you are quite overweight. You may notice changes in your thighs and buttocks, as those are the areas where fat will collect first.

In your forties, though, you'll start to see a softening of your lower abdomen, where there are fewer muscles below the belly button than above it to support the area. This is a result of yellow fat accumulating intra-abdominally.

The abdomen is constructed with different layers of muscles; the transversus abdominis goes horizontally across the abdomen and keeps the bulge of the internal organs looking flat—but only if it's tight. In addition, the area above the belly button is anatomically weak and also prone to bulging. So as your hormones trigger changes to fat placement in your body, any anatomically weak areas will be visible unless special attention is paid to compensate for nature's bad joke on female anatomy.

CHANGES TO YOUR HORMONES

Fortunately, when it comes to hormones and their effect on your fat, your thirties are likely to be pretty much the same as your twenties. The big difference will be that your fertility will start to decline precipitously after the age of around thirty-five. And, obviously, if you're having children, your pregnancies will cause monumental shifts in hormone production.

Like most women, you'll start noticing perimenopausal symptoms in your forties. You can blame this on declining levels of estrogen and progesterone, particularly when you find yourself wide-awake in the middle of the night due to unplanned and unwanted mood swings and hot flashes (the first one of these can be an extremely unwelcome shock). Or when you wonder why your skin is breaking out even as your period is becoming irregular, or why your pants don't fit even though you're eating the same way you have since you graduated from college. Among these and other symptoms, estrogen and progesterone are also signaling the fat in your body to shift around where it's least wanted.

In your thirties, your energy levels should still be strong and your metabolism pretty much unchanged from your twenties. In your forties, your metabolism starts a very gradual slowdown. You might realize that the five pounds you could have easily lost only a few years ago simply won't budge. And if you haven't been taking good care of yourself by eating well and exercising properly over the years, the forties is the decade where it will all start to catch up with you. Naturally, it will always catch up to you at some point, no matter what, but this will happen much earlier for those who've taken the least amount of care of themselves.

That said, from my experience as a plastic surgeon, I find the forties to be the decade where women are obsessed with everything *but* themselves. (Although many women are having children in their thirties, they're still very active and concerned about their looks.) They're instead taking care of their children, their careers, or both.

CHANGES TO YOUR FACE

The thirties are when faces start to lose their dazzle. They might not be very wrinkled yet, but the skin texture is beginning to change.

In your thirties and forties, the four different zones of your face probably look something like this:

FOREHEAD Since you age from the top down, your forehead will start to show deepening wrinkles when you're in your thirties, as well as show the lines that look like "elevens" between the eyebrows (the glabellar lines).

EYE AREA Crow's-feet will start to appear in the corner of the eyes. The real changes here happen in the forties, when my patients universally say, "I look tired." They look tired because they have bags and deep discoloration around their eyes due to poor skin quality there. Their eyelids may start drooping slightly as well as become more crepey.

CHEEKS This area usually looks good throughout your thirties, but starts losing volume in the upper cheek first. As this fat continues to descend, not only does the entire upper cheekbone area start to look more hollow and gaunt, but all that volume has to go somewhere, and it does. It slides down to your jawline, where it appears as something nobody wants: the jowl!

CENTRAL FACE The central facial zone is the area outlined by the nasolabial folds, which are the lines or folds that extend from the sides of your nostrils down to the corners of your mouth.

Women in their thirties don't usually see many changes around their lips unless they are heavy smokers; these wrinkles start appearing in the forties. This is also when the nasolabial fold area starts to become more pronounced as it becomes segmented from the cheeks.

CHANGES TO YOUR BODY

In your thirties, your fat is starting to slowly shift to your hips and thighs. And because this is the decade when many women have children, you may also have problems with restoring muscle tone to your abdomen after pregnancy. If you're in good shape and eat well, however, you shouldn't be seeing very many changes to your overall body shape other than those produced by pregnancy.

The forties are when changes really start to happen, as your yellow fat moves into the upper arms, around your breasts, and into the buttocks as well as the hips and thighs that you were starting to notice in your thirties.

For both decades, posture is also extremely important, as if you sit with hunched shoulders, you'll automatically look older.

BREASTS Women in their forties will note with dismay that their breasts may not be as firm as they used to be. You might see a redistribution of fat so that there's more volume on the outside, making your breasts look flatter and droop toward your arms when you lie down.

ARMS In your thirties, whatever you do to firm up your arms will show up beautifully, so this is the ideal time to start working with bungee cords and/or light hand weights.

As you enter your forties you'll notice your triceps starting to look a little fleshy-looking and less defined, leading to that dreaded upper-arm sag—what many of my patients call bat wings.

HANDS Your hands should still look good, unless you spend a lot of time in the sun, which will give you age spots, freckles, and a loss of skin elasticity.

BACK Your back should still look good in your thirties and forties.

ABDOMINAL AREA Everyone's abdominal muscles are different; you may have naturally strong obliques (the muscles at the sides of your waist), while your sister may have less definition at her waistline. Like most women of all ages, though, you'll tend to have weak lower abs (unless you're a dancer or do a lot of core-intensive exercise; there are specific exercises for the lower abs in part 3).

In your forties, however, the lower abdominal area will show even more marked changes, as three things happen to create the dreaded "pooch": Weak muscles continue to get weaker; hormonal changes trigger extra fat deposits; and the fat collects in the abdomen and around the intestines, which starts to push the abdomen outward in the weakest area (which is, unfortunately, the lower abdomen).

ABOUT YOUR FASCIA

Every muscle is encased in a layer of tissue called fascia. Muscle on its own doesn't have a structure—that structure is provided by the fascia, which holds your muscles in the proper position next to your bones. You can see what it looks like next time you're cutting a raw chicken; when you take the meat off the bone, that hard stuff that you can't pull is the fascia.

Think of fascia as being like skin, especially since you can actually improve the quality of your fascia with good nutrition and with exercises that increase lean muscle mass. Improper nutrition and lack of movement will stretch your fascia out of shape—and once it does, it will take a long time, perhaps even several months, to snap back.

Healthy fascia also has a better relationship with the muscle itself, so that the muscle will be firmer within the casing of the fascia—creating a shape and contour that looks as it did when you were much younger. This is particularly noticeable in your butt; strengthen the glutes and you'll help support your fascia and keep everything lifted.

Dealing with this abdominal fat is a must—the Eating Plan in part 2 directly targets subcutaneous fat volume, and lower abdominal weakness is reversed with the Core Curriculum program in part 3. When you develop a strong muscular wall, it will keep this area flat despite the internal, hormonally driven changes to fat, and despite the variations in your diet throughout the day.

BUTTOCKS Unfortunately, the gluteal muscles (or glutes) begin to fall when you're in your thirties, and once the skin has been stretched out in the infragluteal fold, where your buttocks meet your thighs, it's a challenge to get it back to the youthful relationship where the lower butt is well demarcated from the back of the thigh, creating the ever-desirable rounded "bubble" look.

Fortunately, you can lessen the drooping and loss of shapeliness by doing focused exercises, as you'll see in part 3.

THIGHS You'll probably retain your flexibility and firm thighs in your thirties, but that's also the time when you begin to deposit more fat, usually in the lateral (outside, or saddlebags) and medial (inside) thighs. These fat deposits will become more pronounced in your forties.

KNEES If you exercise regularly, your knees should look pretty good. If you don't, in your forties they will gradually start to lose definition and become rounded, with pockets of fat on either side of your kneecaps.

CALVES Calves, as a rule, do not collect fat. (Ankles only collect fat with obesity, so they're not applicable to the scope of this book.) The definition of your calves is genetically determined, but since they are comprised of a beautiful diamond-shaped complex of two muscles, when they are well defined, they balance the thighs and make the leg look young.

CHANGES TO YOUR BODY AFTER PREGNANCY

When you have children, your body undergoes some of the most amazing changes you'll ever live through, and it's certainly worth the aching feet, swollen ankles, and humongous belly so you can have a healthy baby. But the nine months of pregnancy also wreak havoc on the fascia and muscles of the abdomen.

As a result, in my practice, most of my patients come to see me after they're done having children. They need my advice because they've tried everything but aren't able to get a flat abdomen despite doing over a hundred crunches a day. At the same time, they can't shed much of their postpregnancy weight, having reached a plateau that simply will not budge. Worse, this weight is found in the areas where soft yellow fat is already prone to collect—in the midsection of the body, the abdomen, buttocks, and thighs. And since added weight in these areas makes a body look "matronly," these patients are distraught about their postpregnancy shape, and are absolutely determined to look sexy and young again. All they talk to me about is the shape of their breasts and the droop of their abdomens, despite their frequent stints doing cardio in the gym and their highly restrictive diets. As a result, they are shredded of body fat, have no volume in their sagging breasts, and have flat but loose-skinned abdomens and thin, gaunt faces that look much older than their chronological ages.

If these complaints sound familiar, the Brown Fat Revolution will give you your body back.

3.
HOW YOU AGE—AND HOW FAT PLAYS ITS ROLE: HORMONE CATEGORY II

Even if you've been diligent about nutrition and fitness all your life, you're going to encounter many new body challenges once you hit fifty and beyond.

It's particularly common for women to tell me they're doing everything "right"—usually this means they are eating and exercising according to a program they picked up in a magazine or at the gym—but they're not getting the results they want.

Many of these women tell me they just want to give up. They don't know what to do anymore because they're finding it so much harder to shift the weight that once would have melted away easily. Conventional diets and workout regimens aren't helping anymore. They don't know where to go for advice, either.

Take Susan. She's always taken care of herself; she doesn't drink or smoke and she stays out of the sun. But since she turned fifty, she tells me, she's suddenly beginning to feel that she looks *old*.

"I'm starting to look like my mother!" she wailed.

I take a good look, and see a very thin woman with dry, lifeless, wrinkled skin. Her cheeks are flat; deep folds run from her nostrils to the corners of her mouth; her lips are thin and pursed; and she has the characteristic 11 wrinkles between her eyebrows. Even more noticeable—Susan's harsh and tired face doesn't match her body, which is mostly still firm and shapely, although there are new bulges in the lower belly, around the folds at the sides of her breasts, and at her flanks.

What happened? In her late thirties, after her children were born, Susan started a regimented low-carb, high-protein diet, coupled with daily workouts. She looked and felt great. But as she approached fifty, her vibrant looks vanished. It never occurred to her that the very lifestyle that had carried her through her forties was now taking its toll, and that her restrictive diet and everyday workouts were literally wearing down her body.

When I told her she should think about changing her diet and exercise routine, she looked at me in shock. But then I explained that it was wrong to think that a very low-carb diet is best—or that cardiovascular exercise is almost infinitely beneficial and can't be overdone. It isn't, and it can. Once she followed my suggestions, she was soon on the road to good health and a more youthful face.

HOW YOU AGE IN YOUR FIFTIES AND OLDER

One thing I've learned after thirty years as a plastic surgeon is that the way a woman in her fifties and older ages comes from many factors. It's not just about wrinkles and age spots and sagging—it's a lot more complex.

Although many women now truly believe that, thanks to wonderful medical advances (like Botox and injectable fillers), "Fifty is the new forty," hitting 5-0 can still be traumatic. While dealing with turning forty might have marked a turning point, going through menopause signals the true end of youth. Getting older and *looking* older causes a potent shift in your emotions. You literally can't pretend you're still young, even if your face is smooth and relatively unlined. And as you move on to this phase of your life, dealing with whatever stress comes your way, it doesn't help when your body seems to be turning against you.

What I hear most often from my patients who are fifty and older is that they've raised their children, they've had either great careers or the satisfying work that comes from rearing a family, and now they're focusing on their own needs. Believe me, they've earned that right. And it's certainly not vanity that makes these women want to look better.

Instead, it's all about dealing with the profound disconnect they feel when they look in the mirror. Inside, they're still young and vibrant and gorgeous. But the outside version looking back at them doesn't match their inner self. When this happens, they worry that they're being judged as frumpy or old when they actually feel pretty great inside—the way they did when they were much younger, made even better since they also have all the wisdom they've accrued from their life experiences.

Fortunately, women in their fifties and up are able to get (and keep) some of the most dramatic results once they stick to my plan, watching in awe as they transform their faces and bodies, by replacing their old yellow fat with nice new, resilient brown fat, and improving their energy and stamina.

If you stick to my plan, within two months you should be a new woman, too. You'll have a tight, toned midsection thanks to all your firm brown fat, as well as straight posture, softer and smoother skin, improved flexibility and strength, and an overall sense of confidence and youth.

CHANGES TO YOUR CELLS

As cells age, they don't work as well or replicate as effectively as they once did. When the epidermis and its underlying layers of collagen and elastin start to contain a critical percentage of senescent cells, the skin is no longer taut and firm. In fact, they can seem to change literally overnight, especially following a vacation in the sun, a divorce, a death, or some other event that puts the body under stress.

Even if you have a healthy lifestyle, this breakdown is still inevitable—which is why you might suddenly start to look, well, *old*!

CHANGES TO YOUR FAT

The most noticeable overall change is likely to be in your overall body shape. If you've been an hourglass or pear shape, you'll gradually see a less defined waist and more of an apple shape, with pronounced belly fat. That's because declining hormone levels lead to more bad yellow fat deposits deep inside your body, particularly around your intestines, and this process accelerates once you turn fifty.

If, like Susan, you react to these changes in your fat placement by overdieting or overexercising or both, your body won't be able to maintain the proper balance of brown fat to yellow fat. Why does this happen? For one thing, cardio exercise has only a minimal effect on internal fat; it primarily strengthens muscles and improves your heart, lungs, and circulation. For another, overdieting shreds your body of all fat and weakens your muscles and fascia. It shuts down your metabolism into starvation mode, causing your body to hoard any calories you do eat—and as soon as you resume normal eating, you'll still have a lowered metabolism, so you'll quickly put on weight since you won't need as many calories each day. And without the support of good, dense brown fat, your face will thin, removing the internal support of already-challenged skin.

As you'll see in chapter 4, the best way to control your fat is by controlling how and when you eat carbohydrates. The Brown Fat Revolution has been designed to remove yellow fat deposits from areas prone to having them; to continuously burn off any excess calories by developing lean muscle mass in the core of your body; and to strategically build muscle strength and definition to minimize any fat that inevitably does deposit, particularly in the abdominal area.

CHANGES TO YOUR HORMONES

Approaching full menopause is a time of tumultuous hormonal change, second only to those teenage years. During puberty the female hormones, most notably estrogen as well as progesterone, increase dramatically. In the fifties the reverse happens.

Menopause is a lengthy process. It begins during perimenopause, which usually starts at some point in a woman's forties, signaling a shift in and lessening of estrogen and progesterone production. You're considered to be in full menopause after at least one year without getting a period.

Some of the most common symptoms during menopause are loss of vigor, hot flashes, reduced skin elasticity and increased dryness, changes in weight and

ABOUT HORMONE REPLACEMENT THERAPY

Hormone replacement therapy (HRT) is a controversial topic. Several extensive studies have shown a small but still frightening increase in the risk of stroke and heart attacks for those who have taken estrogen and progesterone past menopause. Other researchers think these risks have been overstated.

Still, for women with debilitating menopausal symptoms, HRT can be a lifesaver. Extensive information about the pros and cons is available at reputable medical Web sites such as www.obgyn.net, www.webmd.com, www.healthline.com, and www.nih.gov. You need to have frank and detailed discussions with your gynecologist about your options, and whether a course of HRT might be right for you. Some of my patients have told me that they needed to be on HRT for only a short time, at the lowest possible dose, to alleviate symptoms and, as they put it, give them their life back. They've had absolutely no regrets or worries about HRT, and were grateful for the ability to manage their symptoms effectively.

On the other hand, I am extremely ambivalent about HRT because there are well-founded fears that women with an increased risk of breast cancer are worsening their odds when they add more hormones into their bodies. I can also say, categorically, that HRT is not the fountain of youth many women thought it would be.

Bottom line: Have regular checkups at your gynecologist and don't forget your yearly mammogram. Educate yourself about your risk factors. And do your utmost to maintain a healthy weight and healthy body to help you manage your hormones the best you can.

in fat distribution, abdominal bloating, decreased sex drive, altered sleep patterns, lessened concentration ability (some of my patients refer to this as "brain fog"), depression, and thinning of the bones.

The age at which you start seeing perimenopausal symptoms and then move into menopause, as well as how your body behaves during that time, is genetically determined, which means you can't control it. Some women have an early puberty and late menopause; others are the opposite. Some women breeze through these years with few symptoms; they have a gradual shift, maybe put on a few pounds and experience the occasional hot flash. They're the lucky ones, as others are debilitated by profound, life-diminishing physical and emotional issues. There is no way to naturally prevent the body's decreased female hormone output, and taking hormone replacement supplements is the only way to maintain premenopause estrogen levels.

Just to make you feel worse, your metabolism will also slow. The average woman starts losing about one half pound of muscle per year, so your daily calorie burn decreases. For many, it's very likely that you'll be gaining weight in your midsection even though you haven't changed how you eat or how much you exercise. Couple this with a decrease in glycogen needs at the muscular level, and any excess carbohydrates you eat will automatically be shunted into deposits of bad yellow fat.

CHANGES TO YOUR FACE

By the time you reach your fifties, it doesn't matter how thin you are, how much you exercise, or whether you can afford Botox injections every four to six months—you're still going to lose volume in your face. You can blame this not just on fat, but on gravity as well.

This explains why the most frequent comment I get from a new patient in her fifties is "I don't feel like my face is my own anymore. My health is great, but I look terrible."

As you know, the face is made up of four different skin zones. Once you're in your fifties and older, these zones probably look something like this:

FOREHEAD The forehead shows deepening horizontal wrinkles. You'll see prominent "elevens," the two vertical wrinkles between the eyebrows. The entire eyebrow is descending, and the eyes may start to look hooded.

EYE AREA The upper eyelid skin looks wrinkled and excessive (you may notice it's harder to put eyeshadow on), and can be puffy all day as well as crepey. Crow's-feet are deepening, even when you're not squinting or smiling. The lower eyelid shows wrinkles, dark circles, and persistent puffiness, so you look tired. The skin over the temple is discolored or mottled from sun exposure.

CHEEKS The skin in the center of the face shows enlarged pores; fine blood vessels proliferate and can suddenly become visible under the surface; and there is an overall loss of tightness. Jowls are forming, and the line from the corner of the mouth to the jowl (marionette line) is deepening. The jawline is no longer crisp, and fat is collecting underneath, in the jowls.

At the same time, the underlying old yellow fat shifts away from your upper cheek and down toward your jawline, giving less support to the skin of the cheek and creating more adynamic cheek wrinkles. (Wrinkles that form during this decade are different from those that form earlier in life—they're deeper and in new areas like the midcheek.)

CENTRAL FACE There are vertical wrinkles from the upper lip to the nose, into which lipstick bleeds. The lips are smaller and may even look pursed, and you're probably having problems with your teeth and gums (as your jawbones are starting to shrink). The lines from the nostrils to the corners of the mouth (nasolabial lines) are deepening. The corners of the mouth are beginning to droop.

In addition, as the female hormones decline, the male hormones that all women have in small amounts become more predominant. This can cause hair to thin on your head and grow on your face, where it's least wanted. I can't tell you how many of my patients complain about chin hairs that seemingly spring up overnight. (Fortunately, they can be treated with lasers by qualified M.D.s or with depilation or waxing in salons.)

And let's not forget the neck, although many women do until it's noticeably aged and then much harder to treat. The first visible sign of the aging of your neck is the collection of fat immediately underneath the chin, which usually happens during the fifties. During the sixties, the aging process becomes much more evident, with the development of prominent, ropy muscle bands (the platysmal bands), excess skin, and more fat. You're also likely to notice changes to your skin texture, with more crepeyness, as many women forget to diligently protect their necks with sunscreen.

CHANGES TO YOUR BODY

Unlike good brown fat, gravity and declining estrogen levels are not your friends. Without a proactive diet and exercise regimen, you're likely to wonder where your old body went.

But don't despair, as these issues are a completely normal, expected part of

POSTURE IS IMPORTANT, TOO

I often think about posture, as many of my surgeon colleagues have what I call Surgeon's Hump. We tend to hunch over our patients while we work, so if we don't build up our back muscles, we can have some really terrible posture.

Because I assume this hunched-over position in the operating room (and have done so for thirty years), when I took up bodybuilding and became much more conscious of my musculature, I noticed how disproportionate the front of my shoulders were to the rest of my body. To balance this forward tilt, I worked on many different exercises to build up my rear deltoid muscles (the back of my shoulders) and upper back. With this focused training, I noticed a difference very quickly, and have improved my posture tremendously.

Even if you're not a surgeon, if you sit in front of computer or at your desk all day, the risk of a similar muscular imbalance is quite high. Unless you're superconscious of your posture while sitting at a desk, it's all too easy to hunch over and develop a Computer Hump, too. But don't worry—there are plenty of specific exercises to counterbalance this tendency, outlined in part 3.

I've also often seen patients in their fifties and sixties who want me to liposuction the folds of fat that spill over and under their bra lines. I explain to them that the liposuction will remove the fat from that area, but chances are high they won't even notice a difference—because their problem is actually not about the fat per se, but about how their thick skin is draping on their vertically diminished skeleton. Their vertebral bones, or the bones of their spines, have been shrinking due to the normal aging process, and without those sturdy bones to support it the skin appears to have extra folds. In these cases, what will help more than liposuction is good posture.

Strong abdominal and core muscles are the key to good posture, which will be discussed at length in part 3. Standing and sitting tall will always make you look stronger and more lean. It will also automatically lift and improve the shape of your breasts. This is an issue I work with on with my breast-reduction patients, as most of them have spent much of their lives hunched over in a fruitless attempt to hide their breasts, and it's very hard to convince them, even after the surgery, that they can stand tall.

Don't unwittingly age yourself because you're used to slumping. Bad posture will always make you look older. Good posture is *youthful* posture.

the aging process. Even better—optimal nutrition, good skin care, and diligent sun protection will greatly improve your skin. It may not recover all the elasticity of youth, but the right lean-muscle exercises and a healthy diet will drastically impact your face and your body.

Do bear in mind, though, that once you hit your fifties and especially your sixties (and older), these are the decades where regular exercise is the *most* important—far more important than when you were younger—part of maintaining heart and lung health, muscle strength, posture and balance, and stamina. Plus, spending the time to exercise is an automatic stress-buster during the years when you need as much help as possible managing stress.

A FEW WORDS ABOUT PLASTIC SURGERY

Sometimes, no matter how successful you are at transforming your bad yellow fat into good brown fat, and no matter how happy you are with the results, you may still wonder if some additional oomph might be right for you. In addition, there are some body issues that cannot be changed by my Eating and Exercise Plans, no matter how diligent you are in following them, because of genetics.

These issues include the shape of your nose; the shape of your ears; drooping eyelids; genetically determined dark circles under your eyes; the size of your lips; the size of your chin; deep creases and jowls in the face; severely sagging breasts; overly large or extremely small breasts, particularly if they are disproportionate to the rest of your body; asymmetry in breast size or shape; excess, lax skin caused by pregnancies and/or loss of a great deal of weight; and fat deposits in the torso or legs that do not respond to a healthy eating/exercise regimen done over a long period of time.

If you're over fifty and still bothered by any of the above, it might be worth having a conversation with at least one or two plastic surgeons. That way, you can make an informed decision about whether any medical procedures might be right—or wrong—for you.

Let's take a look at what happens as you age, from the top down:

BREASTS Over the years, breasts lose their shape and become droopy. You will also see enlarged breast folds in the upper back and over the bra line. Diet and exercise won't reverse the effects of gravity on your breasts, but good posture will make them appear younger and more attractive.

ARMS Arms become thicker and softer, particularly where skin has lost its elasticity. This is most noticeable in the triceps area on the underside of your upper arm, where jiggly skin can be embarrassingly pronounced.

HANDS Hands are often a dead giveaway of age, as they have very little fat in them. As you naturally lose volume with age, hands can become gaunt and ropy.

BACK The back loses definition and becomes fleshy, with pooches of fat near the rib cage.

ABDOMINAL AREA The waistline expands, giving you less of a defined, curvy shape. The complaint I hear most often is "I'm getting thick around the middle." The abdomen will be more lax and drooping, too.

Once you're over fifty, the abdomen is the most challenging area of the body to rejuvenate, but it *can* be done when you couple the Exercise Plan with the Eating Plan. Together, they create an infrastructure of muscles and an exchange of yellow fat for brown fat that truly *can* make a middle-age abdomen look young, fit, and sexy again. In no other area of the body are the principles of the program so important to follow in order to achieve the results you want.

BUTTOCKS Buttocks are also a source of dismay, as they seem to get larger at the same time as the abdominal area. They also appear to droop with the loss of definition between the lower buttock and the back of the thigh, so you can literally develop what appears to be one continuous structure.

FLANKS Flanks are the area immediately above the waist, at both sides of the lower abdomen. They usually continue onto the back itself, almost to the midline, and are commonly described as love handles. Your flanks are a very significant and distinct area of fat collection viewed from the front and the back, and characteristic of middle age.

THIGHS Thighs become loose, full, and wobbly on the inside as well as fuller on the outside. Small blood vessels tend to appear, too, becoming visible in the front of the thighs and elsewhere in the legs. Cellulite seems to get worse.

KNEES Knees develop pockets of fat and become less bony and defined.

CALVES AND ANKLES Calves and ankles become thicker. Many women find they can't wear boots that used to fit easily.

Now that you understand the pivotal role of fat in defining your face and body, let's move on to the Brown Fat Revolution eating program, where you'll learn proper nutrition for turning yellow fat into brown fat—and look best at any age.

PART II

THE BROWN FAT REVOLUTION EATING PLAN

4.
HOW THE BROWN FAT REVOLUTION EATING PLAN IS DIFFERENT

One of the hallmarks of this book is for you to rethink the way you view how and when and what you eat. I'd say that about 75 percent of how we look is determined by what we put in our mouths. So when I see women committed to a meaningful and regular exercise regimen who have not seen any noticeable changes to their bodies after years of working out, I know it's because they're not eating the right way. It's much more likely that they're either starving themselves or bouncing from one fad diet to another—with predictable (and unwanted) results—and not making any progress toward their goals.

In learning the basics behind my Eating Plan in this chapter, you'll discover why it's not a "diet" in the traditional sense. Instead, you are about to learn how to eat so that you can control your weight, and shape a wonderful new body. The longer you stick to this Eating Plan, the more it will give you the successful results you'll want to see so that you can stay on this program for a lifetime of good health, a young-looking face, and a gorgeous shape.

More than protein or even fat, the average American diet is all about carbohydrates and how we mismanage them. Sure, you can go on a low-carb diet and lose a few pounds quickly, but while you might be temporarily making your tissues thinner, you'll also be leaving them wrinkled, unhealthy, and highly unattractive.

On the other hand, replacing fat with unlimited amounts of the wrong kind of carbohydrates will still cause it to turn into bad yellow fat in your body, leading to weight gain, panic, frustration, and bingeing—the beginning of the yo-yo dieting syndrome.

It's crucial to understand that eating carbohydrates or fat the right way does *not* make you fatter—as long as you eat them at the right time, with the right kind of balance and the right kind of carbohydrates and fat. Manage your carbohydrates properly and you will *not* gain weight. Your glycogen will be perfectly calibrated. It will be depleted on Protein Days and then restored on Carbohydrate Days. In addition, glucose will always remain available should your body need it for quick energy. As a result, you will not deposit yellow fat because your body won't need to store any—it will always get whatever energy it needs from the balance of the foods you will already be eating. Furthermore, your basic metabolic rate, or metabolism, will be constantly elevated because you will have put on more lean muscle mass in your core, so that any fat you do eat will be used to maintain your metabolism—and burned off. Any fat that remains in your metabolically balanced body will be healthy brown fat.

The most important principles of the Eating Plan are:

- You'll eat six times a day to keep your metabolism at an even keel.

- You'll alternate Carb Days with Protein Days.

- One day a week is Choice Day, where you can eat what you want (within reason).

- You'll eat before and after every workout.

- You'll eat a wide variety of foods.

- You will no longer be hungry and tempted to binge.

Stick with the Eating Plan, and say good-bye to that quick-fix, quick-to-fail yo-yo dieting that made you heavier than ever. Instead, you won't feel deprived or rob your tissues of the vital nutrients you need for optimum functioning, mentally and physically. When you're satiated by good food, you'll have energy, you'll think more clearly, and you will not deposit yellow fat all over your body, no matter what your age. You'll be brimming with energy and look younger than you ever dreamed possible.

NUTRITION BASICS

Before you start to think about yellow fat versus brown fat, you need to understand a few simple basics about all the foods you eat.

Basic essential nutrients come in the form of carbohydrates, proteins, or fats. They're all made up of different molecules with different chemical structures.

ABOUT CARBOHYDRATES

Carbohydrates are molecules made up of carbon with attachments on them, which are commonly known as sugars.

The word "carbohydrate" itself defines these important molecules: "carbo" = carbon and "hydrate" = water. Why are they so important? Because these are the molecules that hold water in tissues; without them, tissues shrivel like a raisin. Water in tissues = volume. And volume, as you already know, is what defines a youthful face and shape.

This makes carbohydrates the key to any successful diet.

All significant dietary carbohydrates (with the exception of the lactose in milk) are from plant-based foods: vegetables, fruits, grains, and legumes. Carbohydrates should supply about 50 percent or more of your daily calories, with protein supplying 15–20 percent and fats 30–35 percent. There are different types of carbohydrates, too.

For the purpose of the Eating Plan in this book, you should think of carbohydrates as vegetables, fruit, and grains.

COMPLEX AND SIMPLE, OR GOOD AND BAD, CARBOHYDRATES In addition, there are two categories of carbohydrates: complex and simple. They are not created equal.

Complex carbohydrates are made from the starch found in plants, such as sweet potatoes, vegetables, and grains. Complex carbs are digested slowly, so the sugars they're converted into are released slowly into the bloodstream. As a result, complex carbs supply the energy needed for brain clarity and muscle activity without causing spikes in blood sugar and fat deposits.

Simple carbohydrates are derived from the sugars found in plants and dairy products. The most common of these sugars are sucrose (white table sugar), fructose (fruit juices), lactose (milk), and glucose (corn syrup).

THINK PLUMP: WHY GOOD CARBS PLAY A ROLE IN HOW YOUR FACE AGES

Anyone who eats a good healthy diet, exercises regularly, stays out of the sun, and refrains from smoking is going to have much better skin than someone her age who doesn't do these things. That's pretty much a given.

But what's been left out of the mix (until now) is that if you look *under* the skin, what you'll find there will be in better shape, too. The fat will be dense and brown, and the muscles will be toned and strong.

When you follow my Eating Plan, all the tissues of your face will be plumper because they'll be well hydrated, thanks to good carbohydrates. When you eat the right balance of the proper carbohydrates, you'll maintain tissue health and plumpness.

With good brown fat supporting your facial skin, you're going to see huge improvements in its contour and texture. You'll regain and retain your youthful volume. Your face will regain that lovely plumpness in the cheeks that makes kids' faces so deliciously pinchable.

Simple carbs are digested rapidly, and cause quick spikes (as well as depletion) in blood sugar. I'll discuss this at length starting on page 57, but for now all you need to know is that if there is too much glucose in the bloodstream at any one time—more than is needed for the brain and muscles to function—any excess will be stored as yellow fat.

A sweet potato is a complex carbohydrate; white pasta is a simple carbohydrate. The sweet potato is a "good" carb and the pasta is not. From a dietary point of view, how the insulin in your body responds to a carbohydrate—in other words, how your body processes it and stores it for energy—is what determines whether the carbohydrate is good or bad. Sugars in fruits are simple, but the added fiber in a whole piece of fruit slows digestion so that the glucose is slowly released into the bloodstream, giving time for processing. Fruit juice, on the other hand, contains little fiber, so it immediately causes blood-sugar spikes. In summary:

- Good carbohydrates are vegetables and fruits.

- Bad carbohydrates are anything white, as well as any carbohydrate that leads to overeating, like pasta or white potatoes or white bread.

- In-between carbohydrates are grains and legumes. Whole grains are much better than refined grains, such as white flour or white rice.

- Veggies contain fiber, which takes a long time to digest, so there are no spikes in your blood sugar and no conversion to bad yellow fat. You become satiated more quickly and stay satiated longer. Eat foods without a lot of fiber, though, and it's much harder to stop. Which is why it's easy to eat an entire bag of potato chips or a huge bowlful of pasta and not feel full, but harder to eat an entire bunch of broccoli at one sitting.

ABOUT PROTEINS

Proteins are made of their own building blocks, called amino acids, both nonessential (the proteins the body can make on its own) and essential (the proteins the body must ingest). There are nine essential amino acids; if these are not included in the diet, the body will not be able to make protein efficiently.

Proteins are found all over the body: in muscles, in the connective tissue that holds all tissues together, in your hair, and, most important, with the enzymes that regulate all of the body's chemical reactions.

Given the composition and portion size of most American meals, I'd say we're living in the land of protein—too much protein. The USDA's food pyramid places protein near the top, while complex carbohydrates are at the bottom. Yet the average meal has this erroneously reversed.

While growing children need a lot of protein and fat in addition to carbs for healthy development, adults do not. It may come as a shock that an adult woman actually has a very small protein requirement every day: no more than 15–20 percent of your total daily caloric requirement. This is the equivalent of two palm-sized portions of chicken breast and two eggs. That's it! You certainly do not need to eat protein at every meal, every day of your life.

Eat too much protein and it is stored as—you guessed it!—yellow fat. Your body stores excess calories as fat whether they come as carbs, protein, or fat. And if your body already has enough protein to maintain your muscles, it will convert the excess to fat or excrete it in the form of amino acids. So it's a fallacy to think that you need a lot of protein every day, or that it can't make you fat.

Another problem is that protein does not contain any fiber. While it's true that protein takes a long time to digest, explaining why you might feel full after eating it, this "fullness" isn't the kind of fullness you'll get after eating complex carbohydrates.

The best way to handle protein is by combining it with a carbohydrate; by doing this, you will change the metabolism of the carbohydrate, as the slow-digesting protein will also slow down the carbohydrate's digestion. When this happens, the carb will be slowly released into the bloodstream, your insulin will not spike, and you'll stay full longer. You won't feel hungry again shortly after your meal (as you would if you'd had an insulin spike and decline).

This is why you want your meal to be primarily good carbs and a little bit of protein, which is the basis for much of the cooking in Asia (a lot of carbs, usually rice, and a tiny bit of protein) and in much of Italian cooking, too. With classic Italian recipes, a dish of pasta was not simply eaten on its own. Cooks would add fish or meatballs or a sauce flavored with a bit of meat. So although white pasta is a bad carb, the Italians understood that combining pasta with an equal amount of veggies as the primary ingredients of a dish, adding only a little bit of protein, would make the bad carb less of a bad thing. Which is why eating plain penne pasta, even if whole grain, is not as good for you as eating penne covered with broccoli and peas. You'll have a much lower level of blood sugar elevation with the broccoli-and-peas pasta, as the digestion process takes more energy. You'll burn more calories and your blood sugar won't spike.

ABOUT FATS

Why is fat considered one of the main nutrients we need, along with carbohydrates and protein? In the body, fat gives you energy and insulates you from cold. It provides the essential fatty acids needed to maintain cell membrane structure in all tissues, most crucially in the tissues of your nervous system and in the brain. It also carries the vitamins that regulate your clotting system.

Although fat has these specific functions in your body, it is not the preferred source of energy—which, as you know, is carbohydrates. But you must eat fat not only for these functions but also to support your heart. The question is which kind of fat to eat, as, physiologically, there's good fat and bad fat. (Structurally, you also have yellow fat and brown fat, which are not the same thing as dietary fat.)

Fats are ubiquitous in the foods we eat, but they are not created equal. Hydrogen-carbon bonds in fat make it saturated or unsaturated. The amount of these bonds determines whether the fat is liquid (oil) or solid at room temperature or when refrigerated. The more unsaturated components, the more liquid the fat, and the more flavor it has. Oils that are bad for you have no taste—except the faint tang of grease.

Saturated fat is bad fat, found primarily in animal products like meat and dairy. It clogs arteries, increases cholesterol, and predisposes you to heart disease and stroke. It has no nutritive value, so all it does is hike up the calorie count of any food it's in. And if it's not immediately needed for energy in your body, saturated fat is immediately stored as body fat—as bad yellow fat.

As with grains, the refining or processing of fat makes it even lower than zero on the nutritional scale. The worst kind of processed fat is transfat, which is nothing more than oil that's been hydrogenated, or made solid through a chemical process using hydrogen to increase its shelf life. (Crisco is a transfat; so is the gunk that fast-food French fries are fried in.) Transfats have absolutely no nutritional value. They can't be properly digested and will quickly form yellow fat.

Unsaturated fat is good fat. It comes in the form of monounsaturated fatty acids (MUFAs) and polyunsaturated fatty acids (PUFAs). MUFAs and PUFAs contain oleic acid, an essential fatty acid that helps supply the nutrients needed for the brain, muscles, heart, and nerves to be structurally healthy. They can also lower the bad kind of LDL (low-density lipoproteins) cholesterol while increasing the good kind of HDL (high-density lipoproteins) cholesterol.

There is clear evidence that good fats in your diet will be used well by your body—to help it function and also develop and retain its good brown fat.

ABOUT INSULIN AND GLUCAGON: THE ROLE OF HORMONES, AND HOW THEY REGULATE BLOOD SUGAR

It's not what's in your stomach that determines how and what kind of fat gets deposited in your body—it's what gets *out* of your stomach or intestines and into the bloodstream. If what gets out causes a spike in insulin, you will develop bad yellow fat. And get fat all over, too!

Whenever you eat, your pancreas secretes a hormone called insulin. Insulin is the hormone of digestion responsible for managing all the blood sugar in your body (not white table sugar, but the sugar that's the breakdown of all carbohydrates).

In addition, proteins are broken down in the stomach into amino acids that are then used by your muscles as basic building blocks, as well as by your liver to construct enzymes for chemical reactions all over the body. Fats are broken down into lipids by lipases.

Think of insulin as the gatekeeper of your metabolism. It's also the shepherd of sugar and the distributor of fat.

Carbohydrates are the most important source of energy for your body. Your brain prefers carbs for its thinking processes, and your muscles prefer carbs for quick energy. Fat is also used for energy—but for a different kind of energy. Carbs are for quick energy, and fat is for slow energy, or endurance.

Because proteins are used for the restoration of your muscles, and fat for long-term endurance, your body always prefers not to use them for quick energy (because they are more difficult to mobilize)—but will be forced to if you don't have enough carbs available.

Carbohydrates also break down into smaller sugars: glucose, fructose, and galactose . . . which all bring us back to insulin. The problem with insulin is that it's a shepherd that cannot abide disorder or excess. Once the sugars that your body needs are absorbed and used for energy, insulin's most important role as shepherd is to find a way to get rid of any of the excess sugar that is not immediately needed for energy. It does this by shunting blood sugar somewhere else, and *as* something else.

In other words, any glucose that is not used immediately gets stored in the form of glycogen. Once these glycogen stores become full, any excess is stored as bad yellow fat.

Why do you need to know this? Because the Eating Plan outlined here will enable you to make just the right amount of glycogen, to have it ready and available for instant energy. If you want to lose weight, you need to mobilize this glycogen. Deplete this glycogen, and your body still needs to get energy from something—and that something will be *fat*. And at the same time, your Exercise Plan will give you a core of lean muscle mass that will slowly and steadily burn up any excess yellow fat.

Once your body has adjusted to this program, your glucose will remain in a constant state of equilibrium. If you keep a constant and even concentration of glycogen in your muscles and liver, your body sees itself as being in perfect balance. It has enough energy to function properly, so it doesn't need to store any extra energy for future use. It doesn't see the need to store glucose as fat, or good dietary fat as bad yellow fat—it will use it instead for the cell functions it's meant to provide.

So by managing insulin and keeping your blood sugar on an even keel throughout the day, it becomes extremely unlikely that you'll be able to create more yellow fat. And by increasing lean muscle mass, your body will burn up its stored yellow fat.

EATING PLAN BASICS: HOW IT WORKS

Let me introduce you to the wonderful world of trickery. The kind of trickery that's going to give you the body you've always dreamed of, that makes your body think that the energy it needs will always be available. And if it's tricked into thinking it has endless food, it won't keep any extra energy for the proverbial rainy day. It won't store this extra as bad yellow fat.

So if you want to maintain your weight and control your shape by burning fat while staying energetic and fit, here's how to do it: *Alternate one day of mostly carbohydrates with one day of mostly protein.*

This pattern follows your body's natural carbohydrate/glycogen cycle. You'll keep your hunger at bay by eating on a prescribed schedule, alternating either proteins or carbs. You'll also be eating much more often than you're probably used to, but it will be the right kind of food.

So in an ideal eating situation, which is the Brown Fat Revolution's evenly balanced system of alternating Carb Days with Protein Days, insulin will be evenly secreted in your body. It will no longer spike and leave you hungry an hour after you just ate a huge meal. At the same time, glucagon, the fat-mobilizing hormone, will be acting continuously to get the fat out, too.

On Carb Days, your body will instantly metabolize the pre- and postexercise snacks for energy: energy to exercise and energy to replenish your muscles afterward. The carbs will also replenish the glycogen that was stored in your liver and muscles. Then glucagon will be secreted to mobilize yellow fat to get more energy.

On Protein Days, on the other hand, your body will need to manage the relative lack of carbs. It will still need energy to function well. Without carbs, it will move first to your stored-up glycogen, and then move on to convert your yellow fat into energy. Good-bye, bulges.

In other words, you will both be burning any yellow fat you might have while preventing any new yellow fat from forming. Balancing your glycogen stores prevents any deposits of yellow fat. Increasing your overall metabolism with more lean muscle mass in your core also prevents any deposits of yellow fat. The more lean muscle you have, the higher your metabolism, and the less your body will need to create yellow fat to store for the future. Instead, you will create dense and resilient brown fat. Maintaining a healthy volume of high-quality brown fat will create feminine curves in your body while shaping a young, three-dimensional face.

Even better, one day each week will be Choice Day, where you can eat what you want—within reason, of course!

Choice Day is not only important because it allows you to satisfy cravings, but because this deliberate and clever bit of additional trickery will literally confuse the evenly calibrated system you'll be following the other six days a week. This will help replenish your glycogen and keep your yellow fat burning up and out of your body.

Let's look at the Eating Plan in more detail.

YOU'LL BE EATING FREQUENT MEALS AND SNACKS

What makes you feel hungry? True physiological hunger is a complex series of signals to your brain, signifying that your blood sugar levels have dropped and it's time to refill them in order to replenish your body and deliver the energy it needs to function properly. Psychological hunger, on the other hand, is an emotional, not physical, need to eat. This happens to all of us; my go-to food of choice used to be Mallomars, and now it's chocolate-covered graham crackers. (I guess it's the combination of crunchy and sweet that does it for me.)

Emotional eating can be triggered by stressful situations, or boredom, or unhappiness. Or as a reward for hard work and surviving a tough day at the office or with your family. Or it may just be a bad habit for those who like to put things in their mouths. Managing emotional eating is beyond the scope of this book, but I hope that the constant eating you'll be doing on this plan will help satisfy cravings and urges to eat when your body is not physiologically hungry. After getting used to how often you need to eat every day on the Brown Fat Revolution plan, you really should never again feel that empty, "gotta get something now or else" twinge that drove you to the fridge in the first place.

One thing babies and small children do instinctively is self-regulate when it comes to food. When they're hungry, you know it. And when they're full, they will not eat. When I tell patients and friends that I "eat like a baby" because I need to put food in my body every two to three hours, they usually laugh. But I know that "eating like a baby" is actually what your body needs. Timing your meals is incredibly important, especially since most people don't know that eating only three meals a day is learned behavior. In fact, the roots of this unnatural eating schedule actually go all the way back to the Industrial Revolution, when factory workers weren't as productive if they took time off to eat at their, not their bosses', convenience.

You might be wondering how a surgeon who does regular operations (that often last for hours) can stick to this eating pattern. Well, first of all, I bring my food with me in the morning and make sure I eat between cases. By doing this, I remain mentally alert and totally focused on my job (and don't put on any bad yellow fat, either!). For any operations that take more than three hours, I step out for five minutes, eat a balanced meal, and return to the operating room refreshed, renewed, and physically ready to make the second half of the operation as technically perfect as the first half.

On this Eating Plan, you'll be eating six times each day on both Protein Days and Carb Days, either a meal or a snack with substantial calories in it. Continuous small meals do not necessarily burn more calories, but they will stave off hunger; as a result, your overall calorie intake will decrease. Plus, you'll be much less inclined to any bingeing, because you'll be too full to think about more food! I'll show you exactly when and what to eat so you'll never make any mistakes.

Frankly, it's time to get rid of the concept of breakfast, lunch, and dinner as the preferential way to eat. You just can't stoke your body's furnace if you eat only three meals a day. It *can't be done* if you want to keep your glycogen stores in balance and your blood sugar on an even keel. But frequent mini-meals will trick your body perfectly—and get rid of yellow fat, too!

YOU'LL BE FOLLOWING AN ALTERNATING CYCLE OF PROTEIN DAYS WITH CARBOHYDRATE DAYS

As you'll see on the schedules outlined in the next two chapters, you will follow a four-week cycle of alternating Protein Days with Carb Days, in a very specific prescribed order that changes depending on your age.

You'll start with a Protein Day to deplete glycogen stores. On Carb Days, you'll eat to replenish these glycogen stores. The schedule is perfectly calibrated to keep your body in energy balance, so it no longer feels the frantic need to get sugars out of your bloodstream by converting them into bad yellow fat.

Alternating Protein Days with Carb Days not only tricks your body into getting rid of bad yellow fat, but it helps you stick to the program. If you're craving carbs but it's a Protein Day, you won't have to think about not eating them for another few months as you would on a restrictive fad diet; you can have them the very next day.

YOU'LL BE EATING A WIDE VARIETY OF DIFFERENT FOODS ON PROTEIN DAYS AND CARBOHYDRATE DAYS

On Protein Days you'll be able to eat protein, low-fat dairy products, non-starchy vegetables, and low-carb fruits in moderation, as well as healthy fats and oils.

On Carbohydrate Days you can eat grains, starchy vegetables, high-carbohydrate fruits, and a small amount of protein. Simple carbohydrates like white flour and desserts should be limited, but there will be plenty of substitutions.

Since what you eat will change dramatically from day to day, you'll have far fewer cravings than on any diet where food groups are restricted.

YOU'LL ALWAYS HAVE ONE DAY A WEEK AS CHOICE DAY

On Choice Day, you can eat what you want. Of course, you know that this isn't a license to binge and eat an entire chocolate cake, washed down with several bottles of champagne. You should still strive to eat a normal amount of calories for your body size, which for most women is about 2,000–2,400.

As I've said already, I've never believed in strict, restrictive diets. For one thing, going into any important change in your life (such as overhauling the way you eat) with a philosophy of deprivation is a surefire recipe to fail.

Choice Day works on a psychological basis, because when you start this program you might find that you aren't going to be eating some of your favorite foods as much as you might be used to eating them. But if you're having cravings, it's a lot easier to put off indulging for only a few days than for a few weeks or a few months, as happens with highly restrictive eating plans.

Choice Day can be any day of the week. It doesn't have to be a weekend day. If you have a group dinner with your colleagues after work every Friday, then feel free to have that be Choice Day, for example. Just start your Eating Plan on the day following Choice Day and you'll be fine.

After you have been on the Brown Fat Revolution program for some time, you will surprise yourself by not wanting to make your old unhealthy choices, even on Choice Days. The quality of your food selections will do wonders for your taste buds.

I still clearly remember the first Thanksgiving after I'd been on my program for about eight months. Naturally, this was my Choice Day, and I was planning to make the most of it. As soon as the food appeared, I didn't hold back, arranging the piles—similar to what I'd eaten every year at this time—all over my plate.

Much to my surprise, I could not eat even half of the mashed potatoes. The gravy resembled thick blobs of brown goo. I couldn't even look at a piece of pumpkin pie. As for the mince pie, forget about it!

So this reformed Mallomar junkie can assure you that the longer you stay on the program, the fewer cravings you'll have for junk food or sweets, and the less you'll even need a Choice Day. You'll find that instead of eating a whole dough-nut for breakfast and a candy bar or two when the afternoon munchies hit, you won't be hungry at all for that kind of food anymore. Or you'll have one square of really good chocolate, and that will be more than enough.

As for guilt, well, I don't believe in that when it comes to eating, either. If you go off the Eating Plan, you go off it. Get back on when you're ready. Certainly, don't go looking for the food police or torture yourself with guilt that you took a break.

Because, in truth, Choice Day is not just necessary to allow you the knowl-edge that you can still eat whatever you want one day a week, but to help with the inherent trickery of this Eating Plan.

If you're balancing your insulin levels and stoking your body's furnace per-fectly for six days in a row, your body will literally not know what to do with it-self when you deliberately go off the plan for twenty-four hours. The last thing you want to do, which is what most diets do, is deprive yourself of necessary calories so your body goes into starvation mode and doesn't drop a pound, turn-ing every calorie into bad yellow fat when you do start eating the right amount of calories again. That's why so many women hit some really big plateaus on re-strictive diets. They've tricked their bodies, all right—but in the wrong way, as their metabolisms have literally shut down.

My trickery, on the other hand, is deliberate. Your body, after six days of healthy eating and evenly released insulin and glucagon, won't know what hit it on Choice Day. But because it has already been consistently primed *not* to hold on to any excess calories, it won't hold on to your Choice Day calories, either. It's going to let them all go.

Just as good fat is your friend, so is the good kind of trickery that keeps your body revved up to burn off all that bad yellow fat.

Remember, you're on this program for life. Having one day off each week will do absolutely nothing to destroy the big picture of how you'll be eating.

YOU'LL BE EATING BEFORE AND AFTER EVERY WORKOUT

Many of my patients boast to me about how they've just spent two hours in the gym, working out like maniacs in their cardio classes, usually followed by long classes working their abs and butt, then showering, then going home—all without eating. They're ridiculously proud of their discipline and have gotten used to the gnawing hunger pangs, almost as if they were some bizarre badge of honor.

Not surprisingly, these ladies are not happy with me when I gently suggest that they're actually going to put weight on if they don't eat before or after they work out. They don't understand that what gives you energy before and after exercise is the glycogen that is mobilized from your muscles, *not* from your fat.

Since you want to keep your energy supply in an even balance, modulating fat metabolism with glycogen metabolism, the way to do that is by eating something nutritious that instantly stokes and then replenishes your body's furnace. If you don't replenish these energy stores when they are most needed—like after hard physical exertion—then, when you do finally eat, any calories you do not immediately need will be stored as bad yellow fat.

Whether on a Carb Day or a Protein Day, *always* eat within the first hour after you get up. When you awaken in the morning, your body has not had any nutrients or water for as long as you have been asleep, so it is dehydrated and depleted of immediate energy stores. If you allow your body to think that food is not on the way, it will go into starvation mode and hold on to fat, which as you know is the body's preferential form of energy storage since fat has more calories per gram than carbs or protein.

But as soon as you eat, your body will release insulin, which not only controls blood sugar but opens up the pathways to mobilize fat for energy—an ideal situation to be in before you work out or start the rest of your day.

Whether on a Carb Day or a Protein Day, *always* eat within one hour post-workout, as well. Your muscles are in immediate need of nutrients in the first hour after you work out, because your glycogen stores are depleted after exercise. Without replenishment, your muscles will be not only weak, but unable to optimally proceed through the restoration process. Simple carbs are best, as they are easily processed by your body and get right to your muscles.

In fact, any carbohydrates eaten within an hour after a workout are shunted directly to your muscles, bringing nutrients with them for muscle recovery. Obviously, this means these calories will not be deposited as yellow fat.

On the other hand, if you work out but *don't* eat an immediate postworkout meal to replenish your muscles, your appetite will increase because your body will be craving replenishing nutrients. Worse, you may find that you're gaining weight, as it will be hard not to eat more calories than you need once you do have a meal.

The best foods for pre-exercise meals are easily digestible and not heavy on calories or fat, as you'll see in chapters 5 and 6.

You'll know if you're not replenishing your muscles properly because your workouts will become sluggish. If this happens, take a break from exercise for a few days while sticking to the Eating Plan, and you'll be amazed how quickly your energy will return.

YOU'LL SEE THAT CAFFEINE IS OKAY— AND SO IS A GLASS OF WINE

As I've said already, highly restrictive diets drive me crazy. They put you in starvation mode. They don't teach you good eating habits. They might fool you into thinking they're working for a few weeks, but in the long run, they're going to be more harmful than helpful, and they'll get you stuck on the yo-yo dieting treadmill that is more like the road to frustration.

And many of these highly restrictive diets go on and on about the evils of caffeine. Now, it is true that caffeine is a drug, and that many people drink way more than the recommended daily dose. But it is also highly addictive (and highly delicious), so expecting anyone to go cold turkey and stop their morning drug of choice is not going to smooth the path. Abruptly stopping caffeine is likely to give you headaches and will certainly make you feel crabby and blah. This is not a great mindset for thinking about a new way to eat!

It can take a long time to get the need for caffeine out of your system. If you do want to lower your caffeine intake, start by adding one-quarter decaf to three-quarters of your regular blend. Gradually add more decaf over the course of several weeks, until you're completely decaffeinated. And be aware of how many foods also contain caffeine—you'd be surprised at the large number!

As for wine, having a glass with your evening meal can be one of life's great pleasures. But wine, being made from grapes, is a carbohydrate. Will you lose more weight more quickly if you don't drink at all? Maybe. But there are proven health benefits to a small amount of red wine (no more than one glass per day for women). So you don't need to deprive yourself of the occasional drink.

WHY THE BROWN FAT REVOLUTION EATING PLAN WORKS WHEN OTHER DIET PLANS FAIL

The Brown Fat Revolution's approach to nutrition has three major goals: lose or maintain optimal weight, lose and convert yellow fat to brown fat, and build lean muscle mass. Diets generally fit into categories and the Brown Fat Revolution is basically a "cycling" diet. This refers to the alteration of the intake of carbohydrates on different days. For instance, bodybuilders will have cycles used to build mass and then cycles for shredding down prior to a competition. Indeed, this extreme behavior is not healthy or recommended, but the principle is correct and reflected in multiple cycling diets. I have formulated the Brown Fat Revolution after years of working with my patients to fine-tune the cycling program that produced major improvements in shape while still being healthy, balanced, and easy to follow.

Is it possible to lose yellow fat without exercise, as other diets claims? On a strict diet, your glycogen will be depleted as your body uses up its fat stores for energy. But because nutrients are not available to build healthy tissue while you are getting rid of unwanted fat, you may be fat-less, but you'll also be muscle-less and health-less, sending your body into starvation mode, shredding your muscles, and robbing yourself of the nutrients you need to look and feel good and have the right energy to function, mentally and physically.

There have been several blockbuster diets over the years that promise weight and fat loss without exercise. Let's take a look at the most popular—and why I don't believe they work.

THE LOW-CARB ATKINS NUTRITIONAL APPROACH

In 1972, Dr. Robert Atkins introduced the low-carbohydrate diet or no-carbohydrate diet, and it quickly took off. Yet I rarely see women today using this diet other than for a special event. This is because over the years, it's become evident that this is not a diet for life, but a diet for an event. It can help you take weight off quickly, but not *keep* it off.

Here's how it works: As you know, your body turns carbohydrates into glucose, then stores this as glycogen. Once glycogen stores are filled, any extra glucose is

THROW THE SCALE AWAY

Many of my patients have a love/hate relationship with their scales, and their obsessive weighing can drive them to distraction. They tell me that they hate the scale—but they can't help from getting on it every single day (and more than once, I might add), freaking out big time when they gain a few ounces (or, worse, a few pounds).

And then they can't understand why they may have gained a few pounds even when eating next to nothing and working out like crazy. They can't bear the thought of sticking to their diets one more day, because the scale won't budge. So they give up. After all that suffering they're hungry, miserable, and might even weigh more than when they started.

Your weight will always fluctuate—due to fluid retention, gas (yes, it's gross and makes you look bloated), and female hormones, which account for additional bloating and excess pounds at least once or twice a month. Constant weighing will merely reflect these variations.

Just as you need to embrace the notion that fat is your friend, you need to embrace the notion that "ideal" weight might not be as ideal as you think, and that what counts is *not* the number on the scale. What counts is how your clothes fit, how you feel, how you look, and how firm and curvy you are, shaped by dense, resilient, good brown fat.

The best way to assess your progress is by how your clothing fits—though not its size, because there is no standardization of sizing in this country—since clothing is a good way to notice changes in your shape, rather than weight.

In my experience, patients following the plan notice one common quick change that they find supremely exhilarating: Their jeans get loose! (This is what I call the Jean-O-Meter Test.) So I'd advise you to try on your tightest, most body-defining jeans when you start the program. Then try them on again every two weeks. It won't be long before you'll have to buy new ones.

Focusing only on weight loss will throw you out of whack, especially as you'll usually experience an initial, rapid weight loss on any new diet—although this is only water weight. Losing a few pounds quickly sets up unrealistic expectations, and even more disappointment when things quickly level off. And it may be hard to believe at first that, in fact, once you've lost your yellow fat and are on a maintenance program for life, you may find you are *gaining* weight because your firm, heavier muscles have displaced your blobby old fat. This is the best possible kind of weight to gain.

To prove to you how crazy the number game is, I am five-foot-seven. When I was chubby I weighed 145 pounds. Now, because muscle is heavier than fat (per unit volume), I weigh precisely 175 pounds. Most men my age of this height and weight would be considered overweight. But I certainly am not! Instead, I am rock-solid muscle, and maintain my body fat at 7–8 percent, with no fluctuations.

Waiting for the scale to move is an exercise in frustration and self-chastisement. Obsessing only on the pounds themselves doesn't put you into the mental place you need to be in in order to focus on what will work—which is a healthy plan for life.

What is far more productive than getting on the scale is changing your mindset about your weight. Next time you find yourself talking about how much weight you want to lose, try substituting these phrases instead:

DON'T SAY . . .	INSTEAD, SAY . . .
I want to lose ten pounds.	I want to look better.
I want you to do it for me.	I want to do it for myself.
I want it done now.	I'm on this program for life.
I want to be young again.	I want to feel the best I can right now.
I want to do this for my husband/boyfriend.	I want to do this for myself.
I want to be young forever.	I want to look the best I can no matter what my age.
I want to be more sexually attractive.	I want to project confidence in my body, which is a total turn-on!

stored as fat. But if your carbohydrate intake is very low, your body burns the glycogen stores first, then starts burning fat and protein (your muscles) once your glycogen has run out.

This means you're losing volume in all your tissues, not just fat, which is an extremely unhealthy and unbalanced state called ketosis. The by-products of fat metabolism are called ketones, and the almost-exclusive use of fats for energy produces an abnormally high level of ketone bodies in your blood. This causes damage to the liver, muscles, and kidneys, since only the kidneys can excrete ketones.

Severely cutting carbs triggers what might initially be perceived as a magically quick weight loss for a few days, but not for weeks, months, or years. Sure, it's always good to want to burn fat so you can lose weight, but it is unhealthy to do it all the time. A diet like this literally strips your body of all fat, creating a look that is typically skinny but not youthful. Plus, it's not only extremely monotonous, but it predisposes you to bingeing because the body *needs* carbohydrates.

Your body literally craves carbs; restrict them from your diet for too long, and you'll be unable to stop from overeating them once you put them back on your plate. As a result, you'll increase your caloric intake, leading to weight gain and fat deposits (since you'll rapidly replenish the depleted stores of glycogen in your muscles and liver—what your body was literally craving—and then deposit the remainder as yellow fat).

A low-carb or no-carb eating plan is indeed a *diet* in the true sense of the word: It deprives you of nutrients in an unbalanced and unnatural way. And it plays into the concept of rapid dieting to lose weight, especially for special occasions. But isn't it much healthier and more productive to motivate yourself to look and feel your best not just for a wedding or a high school reunion—but for life?

If you were able to stay on this diet for life, you would become extremely unhealthy. You'd look old, dry, and shriveled, with no fat—brown or yellow—to support your skin or give you the attractive curves that define your feminine beauty. Plus, all of the characteristics of this diet will most certainly lead to the yo-yo dieting syndrome, where weight is rapidly lost, then rapidly regained, then lost again, with a few extra pounds sticking around each cycle. Eventually, you'll find it more and more difficult to return to baseline. And you won't be happy when your skin loses much of its elasticity as weight comes and goes and comes back on again, making your face, breasts, and abdomen sag in a most unwelcome way.

THE LOW-FAT/HIGH-CARB DIET

With this diet you eat almost no fat and get most of your daily calories from complex carbohydrates. As you know, fat has more calories per gram than carbohydrates. So, the logic goes, as you radically lower your fat intake, you reduce your caloric consumption.

This diet works at first because it decreases calories. But over time, weight creeps back on, and high carbohydrate consumption leads to high insulin levels . . . which in turn triggers storage of bad yellow fat, precisely what you *don't* want to happen.

THE FLAT-BELLY DIET

This diet claims that you do not have to do crunches to have a flat abdomen area, and also that you can "lose inches in just four days" or "drop fifteen pounds in thirty-two days."

As you know from *The Brown Fat Revolution*, you can get rid of soft yellow fat in the abdominal area when you stick to my Eating Plan, but you also need a core-targeting workout to shape and contour the youthful abdomen you really want. The synergy of my Eating Plan combined with the Exercise Plan will not only give you quicker results, but it will steer you on the road to a lifetime program, not a quick fix.

Diets target your weight while exercise targets your shape. Diet and exercise are inextricably connected; one won't truly succeed without the other.

FOOD BASICS: YOUR BEST FOOD CHOICES

The food choices here are listed in order of nutritional value, with more nutritious items first, so try to stick to those.

CARBOHYDRATES

GRAINS

BREADS

- Whole wheat or multi-whole-grain breads

- Breads made with unbleached white flour

Tip: Look for multigrain breads, especially those containing sesame, flax, and/or sunflower seeds.

Tip: Read labels carefully. Unless the word "whole" precedes "wheat," it will be made predominantly with regular white flour, along with any other grains. The primary ingredient is always listed first on the label. So you need to check all labels, as many breads touted as "whole-grain" have very little whole grains in them. I once noticed that what I thought was whole-wheat bread was white bread with brown dye.

Tip: Manufacturers also often entice shoppers with the "all natural" tag. Any grain is all natural, but not necessarily a whole grain.

WHOLE GRAINS
- Barley, millet, oats, rye, whole wheat

PASTAS
- Whole-grain wheat pasta

- Other whole-grain pastas: brown rice, Kamut, spelt, quinoa

A FEW WORDS ABOUT BREAKFAST

When many of my patients talk to me about their weight, they often tell me that they know they're doing everything "right," but they still can't lose any pounds. So I always start by asking them what they had for breakfast. Often they'll say, "Well, I had a big glass of fresh-squeezed orange juice and a bagel. But of course I didn't put anything on it. Oh, and a banana."

Well, these are all foods that have some nutritional value—*but not when eaten together if you're trying to get rid of bad yellow fat!*

The problem with the orange juice + bagel + banana breakfast is that it is comprised only of simple carbohydrates, with little fiber. Furthermore, this combination of foods has a high glycemic index, meaning that the foods are rapidly digested to release sugar into the blood, which causes an insulin spike, followed by a rebound effect where you'll feel hungry as soon as the insulin takes effect. Meanwhile, that bagel breakfast is going to be sent right off to glycogen storage—and then turn into bad yellow fat.

A much better breakfast is two scrambled eggs with chives and some delicious whole-grain toast with a smear of butter or olive oil. The slow-digesting protein in the eggs coupled with the complex carbohydrates of the whole grains will make you feel full for a long time. Even though butter isn't my favorite fat, having a small amount is much better than drinking a glass of orange juice, which is pure concentrated sugar with little of the fiber and satiation factor of a fresh, sweet orange.

My favorite breakfast is hot oatmeal. It takes only a few minutes to cook, and it's one of those deeply satisfying foods that "sticks," as it's full of fiber so it takes a long time to digest. Plus, you can tart it up with some spices, or add a few pieces of fruit to it. Some people like to add a bit of peanut or almond butter or a few sprinkles of cheese if they can mix protein with carbs that day.

One of the most nutritious and flavorful forms of oatmeal is steel-cut oats, which look more like pellets than flakes. The only problem with them is that they take a long time to cook, but if you remember to soak them in some water overnight, they'll cook much faster.

By far the least nutritious form of oatmeal is what you get in the instant packets, and this is a shame, as many people who are trying to do the right thing by starting their day with oatmeal are unwittingly eating the wrong food.

These packets often have added sugar and artificial flavors, but the real culprit is the processing. Converting regular oatmeal that needs to be cooked into instant flakes involves a process called refining. The refining process is like strip-mining the most nutritious part of the grain, which is its center, or germ. Grain germs are packed with nutrients; the protein and starch of the grain (the bran and fiber) surround it, and the entire grain is encased in a layer of vitamins and minerals. When refined or processed, the germ, bran, fiber, vitamins, and minerals are removed, leaving only the starch and protein.

This is why any refined grains are off our list of optimal carbs to eat. When you're shopping, look on the labels for "whole" before the name of the grain, as in "whole wheat" versus "wheat."

Also popular for breakfast is cold cereal. Unfortunately, cold cereal is one of those foods that's extremely easy to overeat, even with cereals that are made from whole grains with no added sugar. I am not a big fan unless the amount you eat is kept under control. Be sure to read the labels carefully, and pour out the serving size in a measuring cup so you know exactly how much it is—chances are high that you're unwittingly eating two or three times the recommended serving size.

RICE

- Brown rice

CEREALS

- Whole-grain cereals only, with low or no sugar

VEGETABLES

Veggies are an excellent source of carbs—their value is "even," which means they won't cause your blood-sugar levels to spike the way eating sugar or food made with white flour can. They're great for our health, regulate our bowel movements, and control hunger. You can never eat too many vegetables, so if you're still feeling hungry, reach for a raw or cooked veggie and its high fiber content will always do the trick.

The difference in nutritional content between raw and cooked veggies is very small, so I believe it's more important for you to have veggies you like at hand, raw or cooked, as you'll be much more likely to get used to eating them. I like to cut up a huge bunch of veggies, dump them in a large roasting pan, pour on a little bit of extra-virgin olive oil, stir them up, and cook them in the oven until they're soft and caramelized. The bigger the batch—and even a large batch will still take only a few minutes to cut into chunks—the longer you'll have them around. And throwing some roasted veggies into a soup or other side dish will instantly improve any meal.

VEGETABLES LOADED WITH ANTIOXIDANTS (ANTI-FREE RADICAL) The richer the color, the more loaded the veggie is with antioxidants, which protect against damage caused by free radicals. The best choices are beets, broccoli, brussels sprouts, corn, eggplant, kale, red bell peppers, onion, and spinach.

VEGETABLES LOADED WITH PHYTOCHEMICALS (ANTICANCER) Cruciferous vegetables that are rich in phytochemicals, which are natural cancer-fighting compounds, include broccoli, bok choy, brussels sprouts, cauliflower, cabbage, eggplant, kale, squash, Swiss chard, and turnip.

MAJOR SOURCES OF CARBOHYDRATES: FRUIT

Fruit is as wonderful as veggies, and a scrumptious piece of fruit is a nutrition-packed substitute for sugar-laden desserts. If you're craving sweets, fruit is the best thing you can eat. They're also a good source of carbs, vitamin C, potassium, carotenoids, and fiber.

RECOMMENDED FRUIT CHOICES

- Apricot, apple, avocado, banana, blueberries, cantaloupe, cranberries, guava, grapefruit, grapes, honeydew, kiwi, lemon, lime, mango, orange, papaya, peach, pear, plum, raisins, raspberries, strawberries, tangerine, watermelon

PROTEIN

Protein is the building block of the cells and of all the enzymes of the body, so it's essential for structure and metabolic functioning. But remember, you do not need to eat very much protein each day—no more than 15–20 percent of your daily caloric intake, which is the equivalent of two palm-sized portions of chicken and two eggs.

Keep two things in mind when selecting your protein choice: fresh and lean.

MAJOR SOURCES OF PROTEIN: ANIMAL

POULTRY
- Chicken, turkey

FISH AND SEAFOOD
- White fish (halibut, red snapper, sole, tilapia), oily fish (mackerel, sardines, salmon, tuna), seafood (clam, crab, lobster, oysters, scallops, shrimp)

LEAN RED MEAT
- Beef (lean only), bison, lamb (lean only), pork (lean only)

EGGS
- Free-range fresh, omega-3 added, egg substitute, egg whites

DAIRY*
- Skim or low-fat milk (1 percent), nonfat or low-fat Greek yogurt (probiotic), nonfat or low-fat ricotta, nonfat or low-fat cottage cheese, grating cheeses (such as parmesan), low-fat or full-fat cheeses

MAJOR SOURCES OF PROTEIN: VEGETABLE

SOY
- Soy milk, tempeh, tofu

BEANS AND LEGUMES
- Black, garbanzo, great northern, kidney, lentils, split peas, white

NUTS*
- Almonds, cashews, hazelnuts, macadamias, peanuts, pecans, walnuts

*Dairy products and nuts are primarily sources of protein, but they also contain a small amount of carbohydrates. Both are concentrated sources of calories and fat; eat them in moderation.

FATS

When you're figuring out which fats to eat, all you need to do is eliminate bad fats—saturated fatty acids and all transfats—and replace them with good fats—MUFAs and PUFAs—instead. Your body will follow suit and eliminate bad yellow fat, replacing it with good brown fat.

Hard fats like butter or lard and fake hard fats like margarine should be used sparingly, as they're full of the saturated fatty acids that are not good for you. Stick to fats that are liquid and do not transform to soft solids when in the refrigerator.

MUFAs are found in avocados, canola and olive oil, and nuts (almonds, cashews, peanuts, pistachios, and walnuts).

PUFAs are found in fatty seafood, such as salmon, or in fish-oil supplements.

To lower LDL and total cholesterol, use soy, safflower, and/or sunflower oil.

Chemical bonds in fat make it saturated or unsaturated (hydrogen-carbon bonds).

I believe that the best oil for you is extra-virgin olive oil. It's not only full of antioxidants and extremely flavorful (so a little goes a long way), but is metabolized differently than other oils. As oils are refined, they are stripped of other nu-

IN DEFENSE OF CHEESE

Anyone who loves food can't go to France without coming home with a wonderful new understanding of the delectability of hard and soft cheeses.

But the problem with cheese is that although it's full of calcium and other nutrients, it's also an especially calorie-dense food. An ounce of cheese, which is a small cube or a typical deli slice, is one hundred calories, which isn't bad at all. (The harder the cheese, the fewer the calories; feta and parmesan have less than cheddar or Camembert.) But since cheese has negligible amounts of fiber, it's hard to stop once you start cutting off little nibbles, especially if you're a cheese lover.

So enjoy cheese in moderation. It's a tremendous way to add flavor and a palate-pleasing consistency to many meals, especially when it's melted. It's the perfect way to add the protein element to one of your small meals, such as by melting some mozzarella or cheddar atop a sweet or white potato. You can add small amounts to salads, pastas, meats, or scrambled eggs.

For me, the best way to think of cheese is as a condiment. Use it as you would spices, mustard, vinegar, lemon, or soy sauce (none of which have calories) to dress up your meals of choice. Try not to use it more than once a day or you might get too tempted to eat a lot more of it. (Remember, you can indulge in a lot more cheese on your Choice Day.)

trients, such as vitamin E, magnesium, and potassium. Extra-virgin olive oil is not refined, so it retains its extra nutrients as well as large amounts of oleic acid.

Other oils with a high unsaturated component include olive oil, coconut oil, fish oils (not for cooking), flaxseed oil, sunflower oil, sesame oil, and sunflower oil.

AVOIDING PROCESSED FOOD

GET INTO THE HABIT OF READING LABELS

One bitterly cold, snowy evening last winter, my wife was out with some friends and I got a craving for hot soup. So I went to the cupboard, pulled out a can of tomato soup, glanced at the label, and put the can right back. So much for my nice hot soup.

The problem with that particular brand of soup wasn't just the excessively high amount of sodium. It was all the other stuff—the artificial flavorings and corn syrup (aren't tomatoes sweet enough already?).

Reading labels should be such a regular habit that you'll instinctively

PORTION SIZE

Many diets recommend that you count calories and measure your food, but I think that's a recipe for failure. Eating should not be considered a measured science; if you're forced to approach food that way, how and when and what you eat becomes boring and unappealing. It's more important to focus on overall *portion control* and to choose good *quality* foods.

Your body will always respond properly when you eat small portions of unprocessed food. The nutrients will be metabolized and used for energy. But when overloaded with too much food, too many calories, or junk/processed food all at once, your body just can't properly metabolize it. And you know by now what this means—that food will turn into fat. Bad, soft, crummy yellow fat!

So remember, the *quality* of the food you eat in each food group is more important than the number of calories you eat. Appropriate serving sizes are:

- Protein: One palm
- Fruit: One palm
- Vegetables: Two palms
- Healthy fats: Two tablespoons of olive oil each day

One last point: For those moving from Hormone Category I to Hormone Category II, from your forties into your fifties, you will need to slightly decrease your portion sizes, as decreased estrogen levels inevitably slow down your metabolism.

look at them before you buy anything, and know instantly whether the food is nutritionally sound or not. The more you do it, the sooner you'll master the basics so you can quickly scan an item and make a decision about it.

And, believe me, once you start to read labels, you are going to be very surprised at what's actually in the food you buy. Why are there so many ingredients for a simple can or frozen package of something? Take a look at a box of frozen waffles if you don't believe me.

You also need to be hyperaware of portion size. This is always labeled right at the top, but I think our eyes are programmed to skip over it. For instance, you might quickly look at the nutritional information on a package of something sweet and think, hey, that's not so bad. Until you look at the portion size. What you thought was one serving is more likely to be two or three servings.

PROCESSED FOODS TO AVOID

Since processed foods aren't natural and are overloaded with salt and simple carbohydrates, your body gets confused about how to handle them within the normal metabolic pathways. As a result, any food that triggers a large insulin spike will be a food that is prone to getting stored as bad yellow fat.

These are the foods you want to avoid:

ARTIFICIAL FLAVORS, SWEETENERS, COLORS, AND/OR PRESERVATIVES The more chemicals are added to food, the less healthy it becomes, which is why it is a good idea to buy organic foods, if available, as they will not have been grown with chemical pesticides that might have leached into them, and they will have minimal processing. Some additives, such as high fructose corn syrup and artificial sweeteners, may even interfere with weight loss by triggering cravings for sweet foods. Others, like certain food dyes, can trigger hyperactivity in children. So just think natural.

CHIPS Potato chips, corn chips, and other crunchy snacks are little more than fried carbohydrates. No matter what kind, they're not only dense in calories and covered with salt and artificial flavorings, but they deliberately cater to the often-gratifying but self-sabotaging hand-to-mouth habits I know you're trying hard to avoid. Start eating them and it's really hard to stop.

FRUIT JUICE The juice form of a fruit delivers sugar (and no fiber) to your body so rapidly that it will trigger an insulin spike, followed by a dip in blood sugar and increased hunger. Off you go on your way to yellow fat!

It can take eight to ten oranges to make one eight-ounce glass of juice. A whole orange has fiber that helps mitigate the effect of its natural sugar, so it will digest slowly and fill you up. Juice never will, so it's a very good idea to avoid juice altogether.

PROCESSED MEATS Processed meats contain large amounts of sodium, additives such as dyes, and preservatives. Although they will be listed clearly on the label, you don't really need to read it; seeing the word "processed"—

meaning that food has been altered from its natural state—should be enough to dissuade you from purchasing it.

PROTEIN POWDERS AND NUTRITION BARS Walk into any vitamin store and you'll see enormous tubs of protein powders. (Bodybuilders are obsessed by them, almost to the point of becoming cultlike on the subject.) While protein powders are extremely nutritious in small amounts, they are not meant to be substitutes for real food every day. Overuse them, and the high concentration of protein wreaks havoc on your colon because there's no fiber. It's always better to get your protein from real food containing a variety of nutrients.

As for nutrition bars, they're handy to keep around so you can be sure to eat something if you've forgotten your regular food (like a piece of fruit or some veggies) after your workout. But nutrition bars are a bit of a misnomer because they aren't exactly packed with good nutrition—contrary to their powerful marketing claims. They tend to have a lot more calories than most consumers think, which can be a problem if you're eating several a day. Plus, they don't really fill you up the way an apple would.

So while nutrition bars might have a decent balance of carbs and protein, at least on the label, they often contain a lot of hidden ingredients that can sabotage your Eating Plan. (See Sugar Substitutes and Sugar Alcohols, below.)

SUGARS AND SWEETENERS Sugars and sweets (white sugar, brown sugar, sucrose, fructose, corn syrup, corn sweetener, dried cane juice, cane sweeteners, and alcohol) produce, as you know, a rapid elevation of glucose into the blood. Insulin then spikes to normalize your blood sugar and move the glucose into your tissues. If the glycogen stores there are already full, it's already on its way to becoming yellow fat. (Yes, the process happens that quickly.)

The most effective approach if you are trying to lose weight—and using our program to define not just the quantity but the *quality* of fat in your body—is to avoid sugars and alcohol completely. Sugars and alcohol are highly refined, simple carbohydrates that are instantly absorbed (whereas complex carbohydrates need time to be digested) and are nearly identical, biochemically.

SUGAR SUBSTITUTES AND SUGAR ALCOHOLS

Sugar substitutes (saccharin, sucralose, Neotame, acesulfame potassium, Cyclamate, and all other artificial or synthetically produced sweeteners) and sugar alcohols (xylitol and sorbitol) are the kind of fake "sugars" that your body doesn't

THE LEAST NUTRITIOUS FOODS IN THE SUPERMARKET

In addition to the processed foods already listed, these items are loaded with sugar and/or high fructose corn syrup, refined white flour, transfats, sodium, additives, and/or other nonnutritious ingredients:

100 percent natural granola, oats, honey, and raisins

Baked goods (cakes, cinnamon rolls, Danish, doughnuts, etc.)

Bologna

Condensed soups (regular, not low-sodium)

Cured meat (bacon, hot dogs, sausage)

Fettuccini Alfredo sauce or frozen entrées

Fried chicken frozen entrées

French fries

Frozen potpies

Imitation fruit drinks that aren't 100 percent juice

Nondairy toppings and creamer

Pork rinds

Processed cheese that squirts from a can

Snack cakes

Toaster pastries

White bread

Yogurt-covered raisins

know how to process. They have little or no energy value, and I seriously discourage their use as several studies have shown that regular use can lead to overall weight gain. This is the "drink diet soda but can't lose weight" paradox.

Fake sugar confuses your insulin/ glucose control mechanism—and you know what that means: a greater likelihood to pile on the yellow fat. Simply put, whenever you eat something sweet, your body automatically thinks it's really sugar, whether it is or not. Insulin is secreted in response to the "sugar." But there's no sugar there, so there's no glucose to shunt to your tissues. Instead, because there's an insulin spike but no real sugar to manage, your body will tip into hypoglycemia (low blood sugar). In fact, after the high peak is reached, your insulin usually drops *lower* than what it was prior to the spike. This makes you very hungry. It's a *gain*-weight situation.

What you want is a *lose*-weight situation. Trick your body into thinking that it's full all the time—keep your insulin levels even by managing your carbohydrates (with a glycogen-depletion or Protein Day followed by a glycogen-restoration or Carb Day)—and you *will* lose those pounds.

Again, it may be hard to believe, but once you've adjusted to this Eating Plan, you will lose your taste for sweets. Your taste buds will become extremely sensitive and discriminating, and sweet things you once craved will strike you as so impossibly sugary that you'll no longer want to eat them.

MANAGING YOUR CRAVINGS

IDENTIFY YOUR TRIGGER/REWARD FOODS

Many people crave sweets, while others prefer savory, salty, and/or crunchy foods. It's important to identify what your trigger/reward food is, because if you have it at hand it can be very hard to resist, particularly when something happens that makes you want to reach for food for comfort. If you know what the food is, and what needs it satisfies, then it's much easier to find a healthy replacement.

If you do have a specific trigger food and plan to enjoy it on Choice Day—which you should, of course!—then buy the very best quality of the food you can. You will be able to savor the complex and delicious flavors, and you will also tend to eat less because the small amount you do eat is so satisfying. Which is why eating one piece of superior chocolate will be more delectable than eating a large bar of crummy chocolate that's mostly emulsified oil and not very much cocoa butter.

INSTEAD OF . . .	EAT . . .
Candy, in small pieces	Blueberries, cherries, grape tomatoes, grapes, small chunks of peach or plum, small chunks of roasted beets
Chocolate bar	Small piece of top-quality dark chocolate
Chocolate peanut-butter cups	Slices of green apple with peanut butter
Hard candy	Sugarless hard candy
Ice cream	Frozen banana
Instant oatmeal	Steel-cut or regular oatmeal
Juice	Water with a squeeze of orange, lemon, or lime
Pasta (white-flour)	Whole-grain pasta or whole grains
Potato chips	Edamame with sea salt
Pudding	Chunky, unsweetened applesauce
Soda	Club soda or carbonated mineral water with lemon or lime

INSTEAD OF . . .	EAT . . .
White potatoes	Sweet potatoes, roasted squash
White rice	Brown rice, spelt, quinoa, millet

GETTING RID OF SUGAR CRAVINGS

It may be extremely hard to believe, and it may take several weeks to accomplish, but you can get rid of sugar cravings. Once you do, you are going to look back in amazement at what you no longer desire, and wonder why it played such an important part in your daily eating.

Here are my favorite tricks.

Drink water like crazy. Add a splash of lemon or lime if you want flavor.

Cut back on caffeine, which in large doses can interfere with insulin balance. This doesn't mean you have to give up your morning cup entirely—just that you should pay attention to how many cups you drink each day. Plus, it's way too easy to stop at a coffee shop with friends and get a latte that's loaded with saturated fat and as many calories as your entire lunch (whereas a cup of black coffee is almost calorie-free). If you can't drink coffee without some kind of sweetener in it, try stevia (found in health-food stores), which is superconcentrated sugar so you'll use less.

If you start keeping track of how much coffee you do drink, you might be surprised at the amount of caffeine you're actually taking in.

Maintain good portion control. When you eat large quantities of food, your insulin will spike, and when it crashes you'll go into reactive hypoglycemia (low blood sugar), which triggers hunger that is much harder to control.

Avoid starches with high sugar content, like white potatoes, white rice, and white-flour pasta.

Eat sweet veggies, like grape tomatoes or red peppers.

Eat every two to three hours, especially within an hour before and after workouts.

Consider taking supplements of L-glutamine, biotin, and chromium. (For doses, see the table on page 114 in chapter 5.) L-glutamine is a natural food substance and the most abundant amino acid in our bodies. It serves many critical purposes: It stabilizes mental functions, keeps us calm yet alert, and promotes good digestion. L-glutamine also helps prevent the brain from recognizing hypoglycemia as a "crisis" that will make you uncontrollably hungry.

Several studies have shown that biotin, a B vitamin, helps in the metabolism of carbohydrates, fats, and proteins. It is abundantly found in bananas, cauliflower, carrots, egg yolks, mushrooms, and salmon, most of which are also negative-calorie foods, which means it takes more calories to digest them than they contain. Biotin also helps stabilize blood sugar in people with high or low blood sugar problems.

There are conflicting studies about whether Americans ingest enough chromium, even though it's critical for keeping blood sugar stable and directly prevents cravings for carbohydrates. Chromium is abundant in certain foods, including mushrooms, peanuts, and whole grains. So I always grab a very small handful of dry roasted peanuts when I get sugar cravings, and that usually does the trick.

HEALTHY SNACK FOODS

On some days you might be trying your best to follow the schedule and tell yourself you shouldn't be hungry—but you really are. What should you do?

Eat your veggies. The trick is having them on hand, so that when any cravings come, you won't be tempted by junk instead. You will be satiated and you won't gain any weight. Veggies can *never* make you fat.

This is especially important during the day, if you work outside the home. It's easy enough to control what food you have in your house and when you eat it, but when you are out at work, faced with coworkers who bring in tempting treats (and who might not be so invested in helping you stick to your Eating Plan), and with the stress of managing a busy day, eating well can be tough. So you can help yourself tremendously if you get into the veggie habit and have something to munch on so you won't be tempted by the wrong kind of eating.

For instance, when I finish office hours, I often really need a snack. A long workday means my body needs fuel. But it's too soon to eat dinner. So what I like to eat is a big fat sweet potato (not a white potato). It's one of the most satisfying snacks there is, with a slow release of blood sugar, no fat, and a lot of fiber and other nutrients. I always keep a few roasted sweet potatoes in the fridge at work so I can heat one up in the microwave, top it with a few spices or a squeeze of lemon, and enjoy. Cubes of sweet potatoes also mix well with tuna, salmon, or roast chicken for an instant salad. (I'll also keep a sweet potato in a lunch bag in my gym bag for that postworkout carb meal.)

My office is filled with other snack foods so I never have to worry about not having something around to nosh on when I need to eat. Here are some of my favorites:

- Single-size (three-ounce) pouches of tuna packed in water. This way, you don't have to mess with a can opener and you're getting the right amount of protein per serving.

- Packets of unsweetened green applesauce. These are available at any grocery or health-food store. Be sure to get the unsweetened brands.

- Pomegranate sauce. This comes in pouches like applesauce at health-food stores or some grocery stores. It's tangy and delicious, and I use it to liven up a packet of tuna or a broiled chicken breast.

- Frozen bananas and grapes. Freezing fruit like this changes the consistency and makes it more like ice cream and candy. It also takes much longer to eat them.

- Green apples. These are an ideal snack food, as they contain almost no sugar and are difficult to digest. They're considered to be a negative-calorie food, since it takes more calories to digest it (100) than the apple contains (80). (Other negative-calorie foods are fresh apricots, cantaloupe, figs, grapefruit, mango, and oranges.)

While a difference of 20 calories might not sound like a lot, if you're eating a green apple every day instead of a red one, that's 140 fewer calories per week, and even fewer over the course of a year. You'll be eating fewer calories as well as satisfying your hunger and your craving to chew on something sweet.

Since they contain so little sugar, green apples are also great to cook in savory dishes, paired with fish or chicken. An old American standby is apples and onions sautéed together. Or they can be cut up and steamed with a little bit of cinnamon for an extremely satisfying dessert. Bring the leftovers to work and that should help with any sugar cravings.

MORE TRICKS TO HELP YOU STICK TO THE PROGRAM

Learning the language of the Brown Fat Revolution is going to take a while. It's like learning a foreign language—at first the words might be hard to decipher, but then suddenly it all makes sense. Give yourself some time to adjust. This is not a race or a short-term diet—this is a plan you can stay on for the rest of your life. Adjust at your own speed. And follow these tips if you need some extra help at first.

As I've discussed already, you should first identify whether your hunger pangs are true physiological hunger, and not emotional hunger. This can be very difficult to do if you're someone (as I was) who just likes to eat, and who gets tremendous satisfaction from the physical act of eating and of moving food from hand to mouth.

If you're having trouble getting used to not constantly putting food in your mouth, try to keep your hands and/or mouth busy. Sipping from a cup of hot green tea might do the trick. Or chewing on a piece of sugarless gum. So can sending e-mails, or cleaning the house (trust me, the smell of cleansers, organic or not, will put you right off the notion of eating!). Ditto with doing your nails, as the smell of nail polish is an appetite suppressant.

You can also try doing some kind of craft that occupies your hands. I've had patients proudly show me their knitting and needlepoint while laughingly telling me that it's almost impossible to eat while you knit. Not only did they get the bodies they wanted, but they made all their Christmas gifts, too!

If none of the above help, use a timer. If you're really feeling hungry while knowing that you're supposed to eat on your schedule in twenty minutes, set a timer for five minutes. See if you can avoid eating and let the feeling pass. If you're still hungry, set the timer again.

Sometimes you might not actually be hungry, but you just want the satisfaction of putting something in your mouth. (This is why snack foods are such big business—they're salty, crunchy, easy to hold, and fun to eat!) When it comes to your next meal, try something that involves a lot of hand-to-mouth satisfaction, like edamame, tiny pieces of crisp veggies, or brown rice balls.

Make healthy hummus- or yogurt-based dips, to be used with veggies, as the act of dipping and then eating can help satisfy crunchy cravings.

Figure out ways to avoid food temptations during the day. This can be tough, as it takes a phenomenal amount of discipline to avoid sweet and junky treats and eat something more nutritious instead. It took me years to do this myself.

If your favorite treat is chocolate, try putting your daily fix of really good, really dark chocolate in the freezer, in small pieces. It'll be very satisfying to let each small piece melt in your mouth.

STAY HYDRATED ALL DAY

Stay hydrated and drink water all day, as it fills you up. Proper hydration is also crucial to the success of your plan, as water is the most basic ingredient needed for a healthy, high-functioning metabolism. In addition, water not only removes waste products from your body via your kidneys, speeding things along when you're well hydrated, but it fills the spaces between and inside all your cells. This gives your skin and muscles a healthy, toned look.

The easiest way to stay hydrated is to keep water at hand. Carry a reusable water bottle around with you (I like stainless steel as it's indestructible and doesn't add any taste to the water), place a bottle in your car, and keep one on your desk. If water is close by, you're much more likely to take sips throughout your day so that you're taking in a minimum of eight eight-ounce glasses in twenty-four hours.

You might want to add a squeeze of natural flavoring—lemon, lime, orange—to your water, which makes it tastier and adds a bit of vitamin C, too. If you like fizzy water, that's okay to drink, as there's no nutritional or metabolic difference between water with or without gas. Although the gas does tend to cause bloating, it can also make you feel more full.

If you simply down a glass of water at every meal and snack, you'll be drinking forty-eight ounces already. Then you'll need to drink only two more eight-ounce cups—perhaps during a workout or while driving or at your desk—to reach your goal of sixty-four ounces per day. And don't forget, coffee and tea count as fluids.

A common misconception is that since caffeine is a diuretic (causing urination), drinking coffee or tea doesn't count as part of your daily fluid intake. But that's not true; your body will only get rid of the fluid it does not need. If you're overhydrated, any caffeine will have a diuretic effect, which is a good thing since your body can't use that fluid anyway. If you're dehydrated, caffeine will not have a diuretic effect.

Regular soda is nothing more than pure sugar water with some flavoring. It should never count as part of your fluid intake because you should never drink it. Its junk value—excessive sugar, gas that causes bloating, chemical preservatives, citric acid that can eat at your tooth enamel, high levels of sodium—outweigh the fact that it contains water. Soda has no nutritional value whatsoever, so it is one of those "food" items that isn't food in any sense, and it really needs to be banned from your life forever (even on Choice Day).

Diet sodas and any artificially sweetened drinks are not recommended, either, as artificial sweeteners, as you learned on pages 77–78, cause an insulin response, then sugar is not delivered, your body produces hypoglycemia and overwhelming cravings for real sugar, you eat the sugar, your insulin spikes . . . and yellow fat is produced. The less "sweet" you put in your body, the less your body will want it.

Juice should be banished, too, as it is full of sugar without the benefits of fiber. Eat a piece of fruit instead.

I don't know when designer water became such a fad, but I think it's ridiculous. Not only are all those plastic bottles terrible for our environment, but you're paying for something that you can get out of the tap for free.

Before you buy any flavored waters, use your savvy label-reading skills, because the calorie count on some of the flavored waters is awfully high—sometimes up to two hundred calories of pure sugar for the bottle. You could eat a large apple *and* a large orange for the same amount of calories, and you'd feel a lot more full.

Make your own designer water by adding a small amount of concentrated pomegranate or cranberry juice, or a few spritzes of orange, lemon, or lime to regular water. Adding a bit of citrus to your water will also aid in fat metabolism by supplying a coenzyme that helps with the mobilization and processing of stored fat.

LET'S TALK ABOUT FOOD

ANYONE CAN COOK

One day I was discussing my Eating Plan with one of my patients, and I happened to tell her that sometimes, when I'm on line at the supermarket, I can't help myself from snooping in the other shoppers' carts. Often I get depressed at seeing carts laden with crummy, processed foods full of salt, sugar, preservatives, additives, chemicals, artificial flavorings, and junk calories. It's almost as if they're buying cans and frozen cartons of yellow fat and eating them every night for dinner.

On the other hand, I can always tell who likes to cook, as their carts are a riot of color: gorgeous green and yellow vegetables and brightly colored fruits, whole chickens to roast, lovely tan grains, multihued dried beans. They won't have more than a few items of precooked or processed foods—nearly everything will be fresh.

Anyway, as I was regaling this patient with my horror at all the junk food that some people buy, she started laughing. "You remind me of the chef in the film *Ratatouille*. You know, the Pixar film about a rat who is a real gourmet and is obsessed with food. My kids love that movie. And the whole premise of it is that anyone can cook."

Well, I told her, anyone *can* cook. And if they don't like to cook, they can still master the microwave. Or get a slow cooker that does all the work for you; they're extremely economical and user-friendly. All you need to do is add some meat, layer vegetables on top, and add different liquids and spices to make a sauce, then turn it on, leave the house for the day, and come home to a scrumptious hot meal. (Slow cookers are also great for anyone who "doesn't like" vegetables, especially picky kids who'll mock-gag at the sight of a broccoli floret—the cooking process dissolves most veggies into the sauce, so you can hide a lot of them and no one will be the wiser.)

Once you understand the very simple basics of cooking, you can't help but improve your relationship with food. (You will also save a tremendous amount of money, as cooking from scratch will always be cheaper than buying pre-cooked or processed foods; a bag of dried beans costs about one-quarter of the canned equivalent.) And the more you cook, the better and the quicker you'll get at it, so you won't even need to follow recipes. You'll go shopping and see what's on special, know what else you have on hand, and figure out how to whip up some delicious meals for yourself and your family.

SPICE IT UP

Once you've cut down on sugar, you're going to experience a particularly wonderful phenomenon—which is the explosion of your taste buds. Everything will taste cleaner, more intense, and more delicious because you'll become much more sensitive to the flavors of real, not artificial, food.

Spices are a wonderful substitute for sugar. They have no calories, but they pack a tremendous punch of flavor. They also raise your metabolism while decreasing cravings by making food more interesting and satisfying. Adding a hint of cinnamon or baking spice will also trick your taste buds into thinking you're eating something sweet.

Be aware, though, of how much salt you use. It's pretty scary how many people are addicted to salt. You'll notice this next time you go to a restaurant—take a look at the other guests, and see how many sprinkle salt on their food without even tasting it.

Salt addiction can be dangerous, as too much sodium can lead to hypertension, which is a serious health problem. It also triggers fluid retention and bloating that can hide your true weight loss and show up as weight gain on the scale. It's hard to have a nice lean abdomen when eating too much salt is making it hard to fit into your favorite jeans.

EATING OUT AND WHILE ON THE ROAD

Traveling can be hell for anyone who sticks to a regular Eating Plan. Unless you go to a fast-food restaurant that posts the calorie counts of its food (which is enough to make me run screaming out the door, as the numbers can be astonishingly high), you have no idea what hidden ingredients might be in your food when you eat out. And if you're traveling on business and are in meetings or in transit during the day, it can become extremely difficult to eat on your regular schedule, too.

When I'm packing for a trip, the food I put in my bags is as important as my clothes and ID. It's inconceivable for me to leave the house without my handy packets of tuna in water, green apples, dry-roasted almonds, some turkey or chicken, bags of brown rice, bananas, oranges, baby carrots, and/or string beans.

My children tell me that this makes me a supernerd, but I'd much rather be a nerd than a growling, starving, crabby traveler, especially as airport delays are pretty much inevitable nowadays—and few airlines feed you hot meals the way they once did. A snack pack of peanuts or a cookie is not going to satisfy your body during a six-hour flight. Even if you don't like sweets or junk food, you're going to eat it anyway if you're very hungry. And then your blood sugar will spike and you'll walk off that plane tired and fed up and even hungrier, which makes you much more likely to binge on an enormous bowl of pasta or a bacon cheeseburger.

As for restaurants, I eat dinner out almost every night, and have found that most restaurants are very receptive to customizing their menus. (Not surprisingly, I never go to fast-food restaurants since I can't find what I want to eat there, and because their meals are rarely customizable.) Before you order, think of the template for your meal: portions of protein, carbs, vegetables, and/or fruits. Then, once you know what to order, the challenge comes in how the food is cooked. Be very specific about this, as chefs are not known for having a light hand with butter and oil and all sorts of delicious ingredients that are calorie-dense.

For example, this is how I ask for my meals to be prepared: steamed vegetables, no sauce; broiled or grilled meats or fish; whole-grain bread and pasta; brown rice; salad with olive oil dressing; fresh fruit. In fact, I'm so specific that I had a card made with my food preferences, which I keep in my wallet and hand to the waiter! It makes life easier for everyone.

Sometimes it can be intimidating to those eating with you when you are so determined and "good." Stick to your choices, and you'll see how tasty food can be when it is cooked simply by a good chef.

Remember, all you can do is try your best, and don't go crazy if you have to modify your Eating Plan if you're on the road or eating out. Choice Day is also an ideal time to have the restaurant meal of your choosing, too.

THIS IS A PROGRAM FOR LIFE, SO IT'S REALLY OKAY TO HAVE REALISTIC EXPECTATIONS

Rethinking how and when and what you eat takes time. It takes a certain amount of discipline. When you try to stick to any food plan that removes some of your favorite foods from daily consumption, you may feel like giving up before you even get started.

So please be kind to yourself and have realistic expectations. Sure, you will be cutting way back on simple sugars (and sure, if you haven't started the plan yet, you probably won't believe that you truly will lose your cravings for them) and junk food. But that doesn't mean you aren't going to want to have a big plate of French fries or a huge hunk of chocolate now and then, and not just on Choice Day.

I heartily recommend going off the plan to celebrate special events. Or nonspecial events. You can't live a life without eating and drinking exactly what you want once in a while. And if you do go off the plan, certainly don't beat yourself up about it! That's one of the reasons diets fail so much of the time. You feel so guilty for straying that you end up eating more because you want to punish yourself.

All I'm trying to say is, if you're going on vacation, enjoy yourself. And once you get back home, tell yourself how much fun you had, and get back up to speed on the program once again.

WHEN WILL I SEE RESULTS?

When my wife started on the Brown Fat Revolution, she quickly lost five pounds in only ten days. And then . . . nothing. Naturally, she was very frustrated, and wondered why she had hit a plateau so early. I had to explain to her that the first few pounds tend to be water weight, so she was really stabilizing her body to get ready for the big weight loss. And that she should be patient. You can't consider yourself as hitting a plateau in a mere ten days. It took my wife three months, and she looks and feels great!

It's impossible to predict how quickly you'll see results, because every woman's body is different. Each has her own rhythm, her own cadence. It's a constant, shifting balance. Some women put on weight easily and some eat a lot and don't gain very much (the lucky few!). Some women have a genetically determined body shape that puts muscle on more easily than those who tend more toward being lean. And, of course, some women might have the exact same weight as their best friend, but have a higher proportion of bad yellow fat in their bodies, so it will take them longer to see truly visible results.

Furthermore, it's very easy for any diet plan to make a lot of promises early on, and put you on a restrictive plan where the pounds come off. But for me, the truth is in the long run. Only a minuscule percentage of those who follow fad diets keep the weight off. And that's what I'm interested in—helping you not only reshape your face and body while improving your health, but also keep that shape and that good health for the rest of your life.

I do think it's fair to say that women who have a lot of weight to lose will see results more quickly than women who don't need to lose as much. By removing all the sugary, fattening foods and then adding an exercise component, these women will lose steadily. They cannot fail to lose if they stick to the plan.

If you're in this category, you'll see an initial quick drop of some pounds, which (as my wife found out) is mostly water weight. Within a few weeks you'll start to see real weight loss, and that should help you remain determined! And then the weight will continue to slowly come off.

In other words, your results will come in three phases: a quick, initial spurt; slower weight loss; then a spurt of greater weight loss until you reach your target.

What's crucial to remember during the middle phase is that although you might think nothing is happening, *it is*. The bad yellow fat that took years to accumulate is gradually being converted to good brown fat. Unfortunately, you can't see this internal shift, although you might feel it as your energy improves.

And then, suddenly, your weight will seem to just disappear once your body approaches a more normal distribution of good brown fat.

If, on the other hand, you're close to your target weight already but are stuck in a weight-loss rut and wondering why nothing you've tried will work, you should lose the weight very quickly. Women in this category tend to be regular exercisers, so when they change gears and really work their core, they'll see visible results in only a few weeks.

No matter what shape you're in when you start, there are rewards at each phase, and you're going to get to see positive changes quite quickly. Your energy level will be better, your skin will look better, you'll sleep better, and your stress management will be better.

Once you're close to your target weight, in the last phase of the program—when your old yellow fat is nearly gone and your brown fat has you looking firm and lean—you'll feel so different and so young, it will be truly unbelievable how different and young you'll feel.

5.
FOUR-WEEK EATING PLAN FOR THE HORMONE CATEGORY I

The Eating Plan schedule is finely calibrated to give you the perfect balance of foods to burn off yellow fat and replace it with good brown fat. It follows a specific pattern of Carb Day, Protein Day, and Choice Day, always starting with a Protein Day to delete your glycogen stores so you won't put on yellow fat.

The seven-day pattern for Hormone Category I is Protein Day, Carb Day, Protein Day, Carb Day, Protein Day, Carb Day, Choice Day.

On each Protein Day you have two carb choices, four protein choices, four vegetable choices, and three to four fruit choices.

On each Carbohydrate Day you have four carb choices, four protein choices, four vegetable choices, and two to three fruit choices.

This pattern is then repeated every week to make up your four-week schedule. You do not need to start your schedule on a Sunday or Monday. It's probably easiest to pick your Choice Day first and work backward from that.

Do your best to stick to the schedule—the more closely you follow it, the more likely you are to see quicker results.

You'll also see that there are two separate schedules, tailored to your workout time. You will not need to work out every day, but on the days that you do, you'll change your eating schedule depending on what time your workout is. Remember to supply your muscles with carbohydrates within both the hour before and the hour after you exercise, whether you are on a Protein, Carb, or Choice Day.

On days when you don't exercise, the only change you need to make to the schedule is to replace the carb in the preworkout and postworkout meal with a vegetable.

Note: Although you know that all grains, vegetables, and fruits are carbohydrates, to make your choices easier to follow, the "carbs" you see in the following lists are grains; veggies (all in the negative-food category) and fruit are listed separately. The high-fiber carbs listed here produce a completely different insulin/blood glucose response to prevent deposits of yellow fat. So yes, you can eat bagels or the occasional muffin made from whole grains, as they are simple carbs that will be rapidly used up by your muscles when you exercise. In fact, you may find that you have a stronger, more focused workout when you are fueled by the right amount of carbs.

TIPS BEFORE YOU START

WHAT IF I MISS A MEAL?

Perhaps you're in a long meeting at work and miss a meal completely. Don't worry—but don't try to catch up with the next meal. Just eat a little earlier and continue from that point to complete the day. *Never* wait until you're starving to eat; by that time, your body is screaming for fuel. If you allow yourself to get really hungry, it's very easy to unwittingly overeat.

WHAT IF I'M HUNGRY BETWEEN MEALS?

You might still get hungry between meals while your body is adjusting to this new schedule. This is perfectly normal, so be prepared to manage any cravings; if you allow yourself to get too hungry, it will be harder to make smart food choices. Don't worry if it takes a while to undo old habits, particularly if you've tended to snack often. Just grab those veggies!

- On Protein Days, you can eat any nonstarchy vegetable, such as broccoli or spinach.

- On Carb Days, you can eat any vegetable, including starchy veggies like potatoes.

- The size of the snack should be no larger than a closed fist.

WILL I GET BLOATED FROM ALL THE ROUGHAGE?

Many of my patients have told me that as soon as they go on any diet, they get severely bloated. You should not have this problem on the Brown Fat Revolution plan, which is designed to balance the digestive process.

Healthy colonies of lactobacteria in the colon guard against bloating and irregular or foul-smelling (poorly digested) bowel movements. These colonies are depleted whenever you eat excessive quantities of sweets, sugars, and/or white carbs; imbibe excessive amounts of alcohol; or take a course of antibiotics, which kills off the good bacteria in the intestines along with the bad ones that gave you an infection.

If, however, you cut way down on sugar as well as incorporate dietary fiber, nonstarchy vegetables, and probiotic yogurt into your diet, you will promote the growth of the good bacteria colonies. In addition, any problems with constipation ought to be lessened, if not disappear altogether. You should have more regular, normal bowel movements. The better the diet, the better your elimination, and the less bloating there will be.

EATING SCHEDULES IF YOU WORK OUT IN THE MORNING*

If you get up earlier or later than 7 A.M., adjust the schedule accordingly.

PROTEIN DAY

MEAL #1/WAKE UP (PREWORKOUT)

7–8 A.M.
1 protein
1 carb
8 ounces water
Coffee (half caffeine/half decaf) or tea

WORKOUT

8–9 A.M.
8 ounces water

MEAL #2/POSTWORKOUT

9–10 A.M.
1 carb
1 fruit
8 ounces water

MEAL #3/LUNCH

12–1 P.M.
1 protein
2 vegetables
8 ounces water

MEAL #4/MIDAFTERNOON

3–4 P.M.
1 fruit
8 ounces water

*Note: If no portion size is specified, use an amount of food no bigger than a closed fist. And don't forget, you should drink at least 8 ounces of water with all meals and snacks.

MEAL #5/DINNER

6–7 P.M.
1 protein
2 vegetables
8 ounces water

MEAL #6/EVENING

9–11 P.M.
1 protein, with or without fruit
8 ounces water

PROTEIN DAY
(WITH FIVE SUGGESTED FOOD CHOICES FOR EACH MEAL)

MEAL #1/WAKE UP (PREWORKOUT)

7–8 A.M.
1. 2 poached eggs served over toasted whole-wheat English muffin. Coffee (half caffeine/half decaf) or tea.

2. Chocolate Chip French Toast: Beat 2 egg whites with 1 tablespoon low-fat milk and 4 teaspoons semisweet chocolate chips. Dip 2 slices of whole-wheat toast or multigrain bread in mixture and brown on both sides in a skillet that has been lightly coated with vegetable spray. Serve with 2 teaspoons all-fruit sugar-free jam (optional) or sprinkle with cinnamon. Coffee (half caffeine/half decaf) or tea.

3. 1 serving cooked oatmeal served with 1 cup soy milk. Coffee (half caffeine/half decaf) or tea.

4. 1 cup Greek-style yogurt mixed with 1 cup whole-grain cereal (cold) such as All-Bran or Bran Buds. Coffee (half caffeine/half decaf) or tea.

5. Easy Breakfast Burrito: Scramble 2 egg whites and 1 tablespoon grated low-fat cheddar cheese together in a skillet that has been coated with vegetable spray. Season with a dash of onion powder, if desired. Fold egg-white mixture into a whole-wheat high-fiber flour tortilla (6").

Add 1 tablespoon salsa (optional). Fold sides of tortilla to cover both ends of the filling. Coffee (half caffeine/half decaf) or tea.

WORKOUT

8–9 A.M.   8 ounces water

MEAL #2/POSTWORKOUT

9–10 A.M.   **WORKOUT DAY**

1. 1 serving cooked oat bran, 1 cup blueberries.

2. 1 whole-grain bagel, 1 cup strawberries.

3. 1 slice multigrain toast, ¼ cantaloupe.

4. Whole-wheat crackers, spread with 2 teaspoons almond butter; 1 nectarine.

5. 2 slices multigrain or whole-wheat toast, 1 cup blackberries.

NONWORKOUT DAY

1. 1 cup baby carrots, 1 sliced Granny Smith apple.

2. 1 cup grape tomatoes; Fruit Compote: ½ fresh peach, sliced, with ½ cup raspberries.

3. Fruit and Veggie Salad: Combine 2 cups dark leafy green, ¼ cup julienne carrots, and 1 cup sliced fresh strawberries. Drizzle salad with 1 tablespoon olive oil mixed with 2 tablespoons balsamic vinegar.

4. Raw veggies (cauliflower, broccoli, red bell peppers), chopped; ½ grapefruit.

5. Raspberry-Spinach Salad: Combine 2 cups baby spinach and 1 cup raspberries. Drizzle salad with 1 tablespoon extra-virgin olive oil or canola oil mixed with 2 tablespoons balsamic vinegar.

MEAL #3/LUNCH

12–1 P.M.
1. Grilled chicken breast, 8 steamed asparagus spears, 1 cup steamed yellow (summer) squash.

2. Quick Vegetarian Chili: Cook together until veggies are soft and well mixed: 1 cup kidney beans, ½ cup chopped onion, ½ cup chopped tomato, ½ cup sugar-free tomato sauce, 1 teaspoon chili powder.

3. Tuna Salad: 2 cups dark leafy lettuce, 1 chopped tomato, ¼ cup chopped onions. Top veggies with tuna. Drizzle salad with 1 tablespoon extra-virgin olive oil or canola oil mixed with 2 tablespoons red-wine vinegar.

4. 1 cup grilled eggplant and 1 cup roasted red bell peppers, topped with 1 serving low-fat mozzarella cheese (melted).

5. Shrimp Cocktail: Boiled shrimp and cocktail sauce. 2 cups of tossed salad (dark green leafy vegetables mixed with choice of salad veggies—onions, tomatoes, bell peppers, cucumbers, etc.). Drizzle salad with 1 tablespoon olive, flaxseed, or other allowed oil mixed with 2 tablespoons red-wine vinegar.

MEAL #4/MIDAFTERNOON

3–4 P.M.
1. Granny Smith apple.

2. 1 cup fresh berries, any type.

3. ¼ melon (such as cantaloupe or casaba).

4. 1 peach or nectarine.

5. ½ grapefruit.

MEAL #5/DINNER

6–7 p.m.
1. Grilled steak, 2 cups of tossed salad (dark green leafy vegetables mixed with choice of salad veggies—onions,

tomatoes, bell peppers, cucumbers, etc.). Drizzle salad with 1 tablespoon extra-virgin olive, flaxseed, or other allowed oil mixed with 2 tablespoons red-wine vinegar.

2. Baked pork chop, cooked carrots, steamed broccoli.

3. Lean turkey burger, grilled or broiled; stewed tomatoes; steamed zucchini.

4. Scallop-Veggie Kebabs: In a medium-size glass bowl combine 2 tablespoons lemon juice, ¼ teaspoon chopped fresh garlic, and 2 teaspoons Dijon mustard. Add about 4 to 5 medium-size scallops, 3 to 4 cherry tomatoes, and 1 yellow pepper, cut into chunks. Toss gently to coat, and let marinate in refrigerator for 30 minutes. Thread scallops and vegetables alternately onto skewers. Spray lightly with olive oil–flavored cooking spray. Broil or grill over medium heat for 5–6 minutes, turning once, until scallops are firm.

5. Grilled chicken served with pomegranate sauce, steamed green beans (topped with 1 tablespoon chopped or slivered almonds), and sliced tomato-basil salad (slice 1 tomato and top with 3 shredded basil leaves; drizzle with 1 tablespoon extra-virgin olive oil).

MEAL #6/EVENING

9–11 P.M.

1. I handful of almonds or pistachios with optional low-carb fruit.*

2. 2 hard-boiled eggs with optional low-carb fruit.*

3. Smoothie: 1 cup soy milk, skim milk, or low-fat milk blended with 1 cup strawberries.

4. 1 cup Greek-style yogurt with 1 cup fresh berries

5. 1 serving low-fat cottage cheese with 1 fresh peach, sliced.

*Low-carb fruits include apricots, berries, Granny Smith apples, grapefruits, melons, nectarines, and peaches.

CARBOHYDRATE DAY

MEAL #1/WAKE UP (PREWORKOUT)

7–8 A.M.   1 protein
1 carb
8 ounces water
1 cup coffee (half caffeine/half decaf) or tea

WORKOUT

8–9 A.M.   8 ounces water

MEAL #2/POSTWORKOUT

9–10 A.M.   1 carb
1 fruit
8 ounces water

MEAL #3/LUNCH

12–1 P.M.   1 protein
1 carb
2 vegetables
8 ounces water

MEAL #4/MIDAFTERNOON

3–4 P.M.   1 fruit
8 ounces water

MEAL #5/DINNER

6–7 P.M.   1 protein
1 carb
2 vegetables
8 ounces water

MEAL #6/EVENING

9–11 P.M.   1 protein, with or without fruit

8 ounces water

CARBOHYDRATE DAY
(WITH FIVE SUGGESTED FOOD CHOICES FOR EACH MEAL)

MEAL #1/WAKE UP (PREWORKOUT)

7–8 A.M.

1. 2 scrambled eggs, 1 cup Cream of Wheat sprinkled with 1 tablespoon chopped walnuts or pecans. Coffee (half caffeine/half decaf) or tea.

2. 2 scrambled egg whites, served with 2 slices multigrain toast. Coffee (half caffeine/half decaf) or tea.

3. 1 cup Greek-style yogurt mixed with 1 serving low-fat, sugar-free granola. Coffee (half caffeine/half decaf) or tea.

4. Breakfast muffin: 1 lean turkey sausage patty served on 1 whole-wheat English muffin. Coffee (half caffeine/half decaf) or tea.

5. 1 multigrain bagel and smoked salmon, garnished with 1 tablespoon capers. Coffee (half caffeine/half decaf) or tea.

WORKOUT

8–9 A.M.   8 ounces water

MEAL #2/POSTWORKOUT

9–10 A.M.

1. 2 slices whole-wheat or multigrain toast, 1 peach.

2. Several whole-grain crackers spread with 2 teaspoons almond butter or natural peanut butter, 1 apple.

3. 1 serving multigrain cereal, 1 cup berries.

4. 1 medium baked sweet potato, topped with ½ cup chunky unsweetened applesauce.

5. 1 cup oatmeal, microwaved with 1 sliced banana.

MEAL #3/LUNCH

12–1 P.M.

1. Veggie Pasta: Heat together 1 cup cooked mixed vegetables and ½ cup fat-free, sugar-free marinara sauce; serve over 1 serving whole-grain pasta. Top with 1 serving low-fat or part-skim mozzarella. 1 cup salad greens, drizzled with 1 tablespoon extra-virgin olive oil or canola oil and 2 tablespoons balsamic vinegar.

2. Salmon Caesar Salad: Combine 2 cups romaine lettuce, ½ cup grape tomatoes, and ¼ cup chopped onion; top with grilled salmon, 1 tablespoon Parmesan cheese, and 2 tablespoons pine nuts. Drizzle with 1 tablespoon extra-virgin olive oil or canola oil and 2 tablespoons balsamic vinegar. 1 whole-grain dinner roll.

3. 1 lean hamburger patty, grilled or broiled, served on a whole-grain hamburger bun. 1 sliced tomato and steamed green beans.

4. Fast & Easy Luncheon Burrito: Wrap 1 serving cooked pinto beans and 1 tablespoon salsa in 1 whole-wheat, high-fiber tortilla. 2 cups of tossed salad (dark green leafy vegetables mixed with choice of salad veggies—onions, tomatoes, bell peppers, cucumbers, etc.). Drizzle salad with 1 tablespoon olive, flaxseed, or other allowed oil mixed with 2 tablespoons red-wine vinegar.

5. Turkey sandwich, made with 1 serving baked turkey, lettuce and tomato slices, 2 slices whole-wheat or rye bread, and 1 tablespoon Dijon mustard. 1 cup baby carrots.

MEAL #4/MIDAFTERNOON

3–4 P.M.

1. 1 cup melon balls.

2. Tropical Fruit Salad: Mix together ⅓ cup chopped papaya, ⅓ cup chopped mango, and ⅓ cup pineapple chunks.

3. 2 small tangerines.

4. 1 banana.

5. 1 cup berries, any type.

MEAL #5/DINNER

6–7 P.M.

1. Grilled salmon, 1 medium sweet potato, steamed green beans, and steamed cauliflower.

2. Baked chicken breast, 1 serving brown rice, 2 cups mixed vegetables topped with grated Parmesan cheese.

3. Restaurant meal: 1 glass red wine, filet mignon, 1 medium baked sweet potato, steamed vegetables, and 1 tossed salad with oil-and-vinegar dressing.

4. Baked white fish with 2 tablespoons of cocktail sauce. 1 serving winter squash (such as butternut or acorn). 1 cup of cole slaw prepared with 1 cup shredded cabbage, 1 tablespoon sunflower oil, 2 tablespoons apple-cider vinegar, and ½ teaspoon caraway seeds. Steamed asparagus or spinach.

5. Asian Stir-fry: Stir-fry 2 cups of Asian vegetables (bean sprouts, water chestnuts, pea pods, onions), diced chicken breast or lean pork, and ¼ cup low-sodium soy sauce in 1 tablespoon sesame oil. Serve over brown rice.

THE BROWN FAT REVOLUTION EATING PLAN

9–11 P.M.

1. 1 handful of walnuts with optional ¼ cup raisins.

2. 1 cup of edamame and optional 1 peach.

3. Banana Smoothie: Blend together 1 cup soy milk, skim milk, or low-fat milk with 1 frozen banana, sliced.

4. 2 wedges of light cheese with optional 1 orange.

5. Ricotta cheese mixed with 1 tablespoon all-fruit, no-sugar jam, spread on slices of apple.

EATING SCHEDULES IF YOU WORK OUT IN THE LATE AFTERNOON OR EVENING

PROTEIN DAY

MEAL #1/WAKE UP

7 A.M.
1 protein
1 fruit
8 ounces water
Coffee (half caffeine/half decaf) or tea

MEAL #2/MIDMORNING

9–10 A.M.
1 fruit
8 ounces water
Coffee (half caffeine/half decaf) or tea, if desired

MEAL #3/LUNCH

12–1 P.M.
1 protein
2 vegetables
8 ounces water

MEAL #4/MIDAFTERNOON (PREWORKOUT)

3–4 P.M.
1 carb
1 fruit
8 ounces water

WORKOUT

5–6 P.M.
8 ounces water

MEAL #5/DINNER (POSTWORKOUT)

6–7 P.M.
1 protein

1 carb

2 vegetables

MEAL #6/EVENING

10–11 P.M.   1 protein, with or without fruit

8 ounces water

PROTEIN DAY

(WITH FIVE SUGGESTED FOOD CHOICES FOR EACH MEAL)

MEAL #1/WAKE UP

7 A.M.

1. Piña Colada Smoothie: Blend together ½ cup skim milk, ½ cup Greek-style yogurt, ½ frozen banana, ½ cup crushed pineapple (juice pack), and ½ teaspoon coconut extract. Coffee (half caffeine/half decaf) or tea.

2. 1 cup Greek-style yogurt, 1 medium plum. Coffee (half caffeine/half decaf) or tea.

3. 2 low-fat cheddar cheese slices, Granny Smith apple. Coffee (half caffeine/half decaf) or tea.

4. Mexican Eggs: Two scrambled eggs topped with 2 tablespoons chunky salsa, 1 orange. Coffee (half caffeine/half decaf) or tea.

5. 2 reduced-fat turkey sausage links, 1 cup blueberries. Coffee (half caffeine/half decaf) or tea.

MEAL #2/MIDMORNING

9–10 A.M.

1. 1 orange, coffee (half caffeine/half decaf) or tea, if desired.

2. 1 cup mixed berries, coffee (half caffeine/half decaf) or tea, if desired.

3. 1 cup of citrus sections: Peel a grapefruit and an orange. Chop the sections and mix together. Coffee (half caffeine/half decaf) or tea, if desired.

4. Frozen Banana Pudding: Cut a banana into slices. Squeeze juice of one lemon over the slices. Freeze overnight. Let slices thaw slightly for about 15 to 20 minutes. Mash the slices or puree using a mixer. Coffee (half caffeine/half decaf) or tea, if desired.

5. Raspberry-Orange Compote: Mix ½ cup raspberries with ½ cup chopped orange sections. Coffee (half caffeine/half decaf) or tea, if desired.

MEAL #3/LUNCH

12–1 P.M.
1. Wedge Salad: Combine ¼ of a head of iceberg lettuce, ⅓ cup reduced-fat blue cheese crumbles, ½ cup grape or cherry tomatoes, 1 tablespoon low-fat bacon crumbles. Drizzle with 1 tablespoon extra-virgin olive oil or canola oil mixed with 2 tablespoons red-wine vinegar.

2. 1 grilled or baked chicken breast, 1 cup of arugula and endive salad, drizzled with 1 tablespoon extra-virgin olive oil or canola oil mixed with red-wine vinegar.

3. South-of-the-Border "Taco-Less Salad": Place ½ cup cooked ground turkey and ¼ cup cooked black beans over a bed of iceberg lettuce. Top with tomato slices, 2 tablespoons grated low-fat cheddar cheese, and 2 tablespoons salsa.

4. Greek Salad: Mix together generous bed of salad greens, ⅓ cup reduced-fat feta cheese, ½ cup chopped red pepper, and ¼ cup chopped black olives. Drizzle with 1 tablespoon extra-virgin olive oil mixed with 2 tablespoons red-wine vinegar.

5. Lettuce Wraps: Chop 1 grilled chicken breast into cubes. Mix with 2 tablespoons each of chopped celery and

chopped onion; 1 tablespoon chopped cashews; and 1 tablespoon sesame oil. Place mixture inside iceberg lettuce leaves and wrap. Serve with sliced tomato on the side.

MEAL #4/MIDAFTERNOON (PREWORKOUT)

3–4 P.M.   **WORKOUT DAY**

1. ¼ wedge of cantaloupe or other seasonal melon, 1 slice toasted whole-grain bread.

2. 1 whole-grain bagel with 1 tablespoon low-sugar strawberry jam (counts as a fruit serving).

3. Whole-wheat crackers spread with 2 teaspoons almond butter or natural peanut butter, 1 apple.

4. 1 serving oatmeal, 1 cup blackberries.

5. 1 slice whole-grain toast; Peach-Blueberry Medley: ½ cup chopped peach drizzled with pureed blueberries (puree ½ cup blueberries in a blender).

NONWORKOUT DAY

1. ¼ wedge of cantaloupe or other seasonal melon and 1 cup sliced red bell peppers.

2. 1 cup strawberries, 1 cup baby carrots.

3. Crunchy Snack Bowl: 1 Granny Smith apple cut into cubes, mixed with 1 cup raw cauliflower, cut into cubes.

4. 1 cup grape tomatoes, 1 medium orange.

5. 1 cup baby carrots, 1 peach.

WORKOUT

5–6 P.M.   8 ounces water

6–7 P.M.

1. 2 lean pork chops, grilled or broiled; 3 small red potatoes,* baked; sliced green peppers and onion, tossed with 1 tablespoon extra-virgin olive oil, or other allowed oil. Bake at 350 degrees until done (about 30 to 40 minutes).

2. Grilled or baked halibut; salad with 2 cups chopped romaine lettuce, 1 cup chopped cucumber, 1 cup chopped tomato with 1 tablespoon extra-virgin olive oil, 2 tablespoons red-wine vinegar, and 1 tablespoon sunflower seeds; ½ cup mashed sweet potato.*

3. Roast beef (tenderloin or eye of the round), cooked carrots, steamed broccoli, 1 medium whole-wheat dinner roll.*

4. Barbecue chicken dinner: baked or grilled chicken breast topped with 2 tablespoons low-sugar or low-carb barbecue sauce; cole slaw (1 cup premixed shredded cabbage mixed with 1 tablespoon flaxseed oil and ½ teaspoon caraway seeds); steamed green beans; and ½ cup cooked corn or corn on the cob (1 ear).*

5. Baked turkey breast; large tossed salad with salad veggies, drizzled with 1 tablespoon extra-virgin olive oil; mashed cauliflower (cook cauliflower until soft; mash with a dash of butter seasoning and garlic powder, plus a tablespoon of skim milk); 1 medium baked sweet potato.*

MEAL #6/EVENING

10–11 P.M.

1. 1 cup low-fat milk, with an optional apple or orange.

2. 2 slices low-fat hard cheese with an optional apple.

3. Deviled Eggs: Remove the yolk from two hard-boiled eggs that have been halved. Mash ¼ avocado with egg yolks

*On your nonworkout days, replace the carb with another nonstarchy vegetable of your choice.

and refill hollowed-out egg whites. Sprinkle tops of deviled eggs with paprika.

4. ¼ cup cottage cheese mixed with an optional sliced peach.

5. 1 cup of Greek-style yogurt mixed with an optional banana, sliced.

CARBOHYDRATE DAY

MEAL #1/WAKE UP

7 A.M.　　1 protein
1 carb
8 ounces water
1 cup coffee (half caffeine/half decaf) or tea

MEAL #2/MIDMORNING

9–10 A.M.　　1 fruit
1 cup coffee (half caffeine/half decaf) or tea, if desired
8 ounces water

MEAL #3/LUNCH

12–1 P.M.　　1 protein
2 vegetables
8 ounces water

MEAL #4/MIDAFTERNOON

3–4 P.M.　　1 carb
1 fruit
8 ounces water

WORKOUT

5–6 P.M.   8 ounces water

MEAL #5/DINNER (POSTWORKOUT)

6–7 P.M.   1 protein
1 carb
2 vegetables
8 ounces water

MEAL #6/EVENING

9–11 P.M.   1 protein, with or without fruit
8 ounces water

CARBOHYDRATE DAY
(WITH FIVE SUGGESTED FOOD CHOICES FOR YOUR MEAL)

MEAL #1/WAKE UP

7 A.M.   1. Cheesy Toast: In a toaster oven, heat 2 slices whole-wheat bread topped with ⅓ cup reduced-fat shredded mozzarella cheese until cheese is slightly melted. Coffee (half caffeine/half decaf) or tea.

2. 1 cup whole-grain Cheerios with 1 cup skim or low-fat milk. Coffee (half caffeine/half decaf) or tea.

3. 2 hard-boiled eggs (sliced), served on 1 toasted whole-grain bagel. Coffee (half caffeine/half decaf) or tea.

4. 1 cup high-fiber flake cereal (such as Fiber One) mixed with 1 cup Greek-style yogurt. Coffee (half caffeine/half decaf) or tea.

5. ½ cup low-fat cottage cheese sprinkled with 2 tablespoons chopped walnuts, 2 slices whole-grain toast. Coffee (half caffeine/half decaf) or tea.

MEAL #2/MIDMORNING

9–10 A.M.

1. 2 small tangerines. Coffee (half caffeine/half decaf) or tea, if desired.

2. 1 cup green or red grapes. Coffee (half caffeine/half decaf) or tea, if desired.

3. 1 banana. Coffee (half caffeine/half decaf) or tea, if desired.

4. 1 nectarine or peach. Coffee (half caffeine/half decaf) or tea, if desired.

5. 1 cup chopped tropical fruit, such as mango, guava, or pineapple. Coffee (half caffeine/half decaf) or tea, if desired.

MEAL #3/LUNCH

12–1 P.M.

1. 5 large grilled or steamed shrimp, ½ cup whole-wheat penne pasta, 1 cup each steamed zucchini and yellow (summer) squash.

2. Turkey Sandwich: Stack 2 slices turkey, 1 slice reduced-fat Swiss cheese, lettuce, and tomato slices on 2 slices pumpernickel or rye bread spread with 1 teaspoon dark mustard; 2 cups salad greens drizzled with 1 tablespoon flaxseed oil or other allowed oil and 2 tablespoons balsamic vinegar.

3. Salad Bar Lunch: Combine 2 cups salad greens, assorted mixed salad vegetables, ½ cup kidney beans (as protein choice), 1 tablespoon sunflower seeds, 1 tablespoon shredded cheese, and 2 tablespoons reduced-fat salad dressing; 4 slices whole-wheat melba toast or 2 medium whole-grain bread sticks.

4. 1 vegetarian burger on whole-wheat hamburger bun with lettuce, tomato, onion slices; 1½ cups baby carrots.

5. Mediterranean Chicken Sandwich: Place grilled chicken breast slices, lettuce, tomato, ¼ peeled sliced avocado, and 1 tablespoon hummus inside one whole-wheat pita pocket; large tossed salad drizzled with 1 tablespoon flaxseed oil or other allowed oil and 2 tablespoons balsamic vinegar.

MEAL #4/MIDAFTERNOON (PREWORKOUT)

3–4 P.M
1. 1 small whole-grain muffin, 1 banana or peach.
2. 1 serving cooked oat bran or oatmeal, 1 pear.
3. 1 medium baked sweet potato topped with ½ cup chunky unsweetened applesauce.
4. Whole-grain crackers, 1 cup green or red grapes.
5. 1 whole-wheat bagel, 1 cup melon balls.

WORKOUT

5–6 P.M   8 ounces water

MEAL #5/DINNER (POSTWORKOUT)

6–7 P.M.
1. Grilled top loin steak; ½ cup garlic mashed potatoes (red potatoes mashed with ¼ to ½ teaspoon chopped or pureed garlic); steamed carrots; and large tossed salad, drizzled with 1 tablespoon flaxseed oil and 2 tablespoons balsamic vinegar.
2. Vegetarian Spaghetti: Top 1 cup cooked spaghetti squash with ½ cup sugar-free marinara sauce, and ⅓ cup grated reduced-fat mozzarella or Parmesan cheese; large tossed salad, drizzled with 1 tablespoon flaxseed oil and 2 tablespoons balsamic vinegar; 1 whole-wheat dinner roll.
3. Sushi: Salmon and/or tuna and rice sushi (or grilled salmon and ½ cup of brown rice if you do not like sushi);

large tossed salad topped with ¼ avocado, drizzled with 1 tablespoon flaxseed oil or other allowed oil and 2 tablespoons balsamic vinegar.

4. Chicken Fajitas: Assemble grilled chicken strips, green pepper strips, and onion slices on two whole-wheat tortillas, with salsa; 1 large sliced tomato, drizzled with extra-virgin olive oil.

5. Vegetarian Chili: Sauté together ¼ cup chopped onion, ½ cup kidney beans, ½ chopped green pepper, 1 cup chopped tomato, and garlic powder, chili powder, and cumin to taste. Serve with ½ cup cooked corn.

MEAL #6/EVENING

9–11 P.M.
1. 2 slices low-fat cheddar cheese with optional pear.

2. Very Berry Shake: 1 cup low-fat milk or skim milk blended with 1 cup frozen unsweetened berries.

3. Banana Smoothie: Blend together ½ cup nonfat fruit yogurt, ½ cup skim milk, and 1 banana.

4. Tuna with optional ½ grapefruit.

5. ½ cup low-fat cottage cheese and optional ¼ cantaloupe or other melon in season.

SUGGESTED SUPPLEMENTS TO HELP INCREASE FAT METABOLISM

This Eating Plan provides so many nutrients in natural abundance that you will not have to overload yourself with daily vitamin, mineral, and countless other expensive supplements. There are, however, several essential supplements—vitamins A and C, and minerals calcium and iron—that are beneficial for your body even when you eat a perfectly balanced diet. Biotin, chromium, L-glutamine, and flaxseed oil and/or fish oils that provide omega-3 fatty acids are also helpful to stoke up your fat-burning metabolic furnace.

You should be able to find a good-quality daily vitamin/mineral supplement containing many of these nutrients, so you'll have fewer pills to manage.

NUTRIENT	DAILY DOSE
Vitamin A	15,000 IU (international units) per day
Vitamin C	500 mg (milligrams)
Calcium	1,200 mg
Iron	8 mg
Biotin	2,500 mcg (micrograms)
Chromium	200 mcg
L-glutamine	500 mcg
Flaxseed oil*	One teaspoon twice daily (mix in salad dressing, oatmeal, protein drinks, yogurt)
Fish oil*	1,000 mg

*If you use 2 teaspoons of flaxseed oil in the food you prepare each day, you do not need to take fish-oil capsules as well. The better brands of organic fish oil have no fishy taste whatsoever.

6.
FOUR-WEEK EATING PLAN FOR THE HORMONE CATEGORY II

What you eat in your fifties is extremely important—possibly more important than it has ever been before. In no other decade will the proper balance of nutrition and exercise so dramatically influence how you slow your aging clock—and affect how you feel and look. The good news is that if you stick to the program, the results will be evident immediately. The bad news is, there isn't much wiggle room.

In the Hormone Category II years, your metabolism will continue to slow down. Add to that declining estrogen and progesterone levels, and the result is hormonally triggered deposits of fat in new areas: the arms, the lower abdomen, the neck, and the outside quadrant of the breasts. Tighter control of carbohydrates and more attention to these areas of the body while exercising can compensate for this shift in fat distribution.

With this Eating Plan, you will burn up your old yellow fat continuously, and still have youthful energy. The way you eat controls your glycogen levels and turns you into a metabolic furnace in which the old yellow fat you've accumulated from years of eating improperly will be metabolized away, and you'll replace it with new, brown fat—the good kind of fat that makes skin and contours look young and shapely. Good-bye, middle-age spread!

In the Hormone Category I years, you alternated Carb Days with Protein Days over six days, with a Choice Day on day seven.

Now that you're in the Hormone Category II years, you'll be following a slightly different pattern of four Protein Days and two Carb Days each week, followed by Choice Day. The pattern is: Protein Day, Carb Day, Protein Day, Protein Day, Carb Day, Protein Day, Choice Day.

On each Protein Day you have two carb choices, four protein choices, four vegetable choices, and either two-three fruit choices.

On each Carbohydrate Day you have four carb choices, four protein choices, four vegetable choices, and two-three fruit choices.

You'll also see that there are two separate schedules, tailored to your workout time. You will not need to work out every day, but on the days that you do, you'll change your eating schedule depending on what time your workout is. Remember to supply your muscles with carbohydrates within both the hour before and the hour after you exercise, whether you are on a Protein, Carb, or Choice Day.

On days when you don't exercise, the only change you need to make to the schedule is to replace the carb in the preworkout and postworkout meal with a vegetable.

Note: Although you know that all grains, vegetables, and fruits are carbohydrates, to make your choices easier to follow, the "carbs" you see in these lists are grains; veggies (all in the negative-food category) and fruit are listed separately. The high-fiber carbs listed here produce a completely different insulin/blood glucose response to prevent deposits of yellow fat. So, yes, you can eat bagels or the occasional muffin made from whole grains, as they are simple carbs that will be rapidly used up by your muscles when you exercise. In fact, you may find that you have a stronger, more focused workout when you are fueled by the right amount of carbs.

EATING SCHEDULES IF YOU WORK OUT IN THE MORNING*

If you get up earlier or later than 7 A.M., adjust the schedule accordingly.

PROTEIN DAY

MEAL #1/WAKE UP (PREWORKOUT)

7–8 A.M.
1 protein
1 carb
8 ounces water
1 cup coffee (half caffeine/half decaf) or tea

WORKOUT

8–9 A.M.
8 ounces water

MEAL #2/POSTWORKOUT

9–10 A.M.
1 carb
1 fruit
8 ounces water

MEAL #3/LUNCH

12–1 P.M.
1 protein
2 vegetables
8 ounces water

MEAL #4/MIDAFTERNOON

3–4 P.M.
1 fruit
8 ounces water

*If no portion size is specified, use an amount of food no bigger than a closed fist. And don't forget, you should drink at least 8 ounces of water with all meals and snacks.

MEAL #5/DINNER

6–7 P.M.
1 protein

2 vegetables

8 ounces water

MEAL #6/EVENING

9–11 P.M.
1 protein

1 fruit

8 ounces water

PROTEIN DAY
(WITH FIVE SUGGESTED FOOD CHOICES FOR EACH MEAL)

MEAL #1/WAKE UP (PREWORKOUT)

7 A.M.
1. Egg Muffin: Assemble 1 poached egg, 1 slice low-fat cheddar cheese on 1 whole-wheat English muffin. Coffee (half caffeine/half decaf) or tea.

2. Mushroom Omelet: Beat 2 eggs with 2 tablespoons sliced mushrooms and cook in a nonstick skillet to form an omelet; 2 slices multigrain bread. Coffee (half caffeine/half decaf) or tea.

3. Two wedges light cream or soft cheese spread on a multigrain bagel. Coffee (half caffeine/half decaf) or tea.

4. 1 cup Greek-style yogurt mixed with 1 serving multigrain cereal (cold). Coffee (half caffeine/half decaf) or tea.

5. Lean Breakfast Danish: Spread low-fat cottage cheese over 2 slices multigrain toast, sprinkle with cinnamon, and place under broiler at medium heat for a few seconds, or until cheese begins to bubble. Coffee (half caffeine/half decaf) or tea.

WORKOUT

8–9 A.M: 8 ounces water

MEAL #2/POSTWORKOUT

9–10 A.M.   **WORKOUT DAY**

1. 2 slices raisin bread, 1 pear.

2. 1 serving oatmeal, 1 cup raspberries.

3. 1 serving multigrain cereal (cold), ¼ cup raisins.

4. 1 whole-wheat high-fiber tortilla filled with banana slices and 1 tablespoon chopped peanuts (for flavor).

5. Whole-wheat crackers and 1 nectarine.

NONWORKOUT DAY

1. 1 cup baby carrots, 1 pear.

2. 1 cup grape tomatoes, 1 cup raspberries or other berries in season.

3. 1 cup chopped raw veggies, ¼ cup raisins.

4. 1 cup chopped red or yellow bell pepper, 1 Granny Smith apple.

5. 1 cup chopped raw cauliflower, 1 nectarine.

MEAL #3/LUNCH

12–1 P.M.   1. Low-fat feta cheese tossed with ½ cup black olives and 1 cup chopped romaine lettuce. Drizzle with 1 tablespoon extra-virgin olive oil or other allowed oil and 2 tablespoons red-wine vinegar.

2. Slices of cold roast beef, steamed carrots, and steamed brussels sprouts.

3. Stuffed Tuna Tomato: Hollow out a large tomato. Mix tomato insides with tuna, 1 tablespoon chopped onion, and 1 tablespoon extra-virgin olive oil. Stuff mixture into tomato and serve on a generous bed of lettuce.

4. Hummus spread on sliced cucumbers and endive.

5. Grilled bison or turkey burger, stewed tomatoes, and steamed asparagus.

MEAL #4/MIDAFTERNOON

3–4 P.M.

1. 2 small plums.

2. ¼ cup dried figs.

3. 1 orange.

4. 1 Granny Smith apple.

5. 1 cup watermelon balls.

MEAL #5/DINNER

6–7 P.M.

1. 2 lean pork chops, grilled or broiled; 1 medium sweet potato; steamed cauliflower.

2. Baked Cornish game hen, skin removed after cooking; steamed broccoli; and steamed yellow (summer) squash.

3. Steak, grilled or broiled; steamed mixed vegetables; tossed salad (salad greens and salad veggies) drizzled with 1 tablespoon extra-virgin olive oil and 2 tablespoons balsamic vinegar.

4. Baked turkey breast, ½ baked acorn squash, and steamed zucchini.

5. Grilled or steamed shrimp, sliced tomato, and steamed broccoli.

MEAL #6/EVENING

9–11 P.M.

1. Yogurt Smoothie: Blend together ½ cup Greek-style yogurt, ½ cup low-fat or skim milk, and 1 frozen banana (sliced).

2. 1 cup soy, low-fat, or skim milk; ¼ cup dried figs or raisins.

3. Handful of almonds or pistachios, 1 apple.

4. 1 serving low-fat string mozzarella cheese, 2 small apricots.

5. 1 serving low-fat cottage cheese, 1 cup grapes.

CARBOHYDRATE DAY

MEAL #1/WAKE UP (PREWORKOUT)

7–8 A.M.
1 protein
1 carb
8 ounces water
1 cup coffee (half caffeine/half decaf) or tea

WORKOUT

8–9 A.M.
8 ounces water

MEAL #2/POSTWORKOUT

9–10 A.M.
1 carb
1 fruit
8 ounces water

MEAL #3/LUNCH

12–1 P.M.
1 protein
1 carb
2 vegetables
8 ounces water

3–4 P.M.   1 fruit
            8 ounces water

MEAL #5/DINNER

6–7 P.M.   1 protein
            1 carb
            2 vegetables
            8 ounces water

MEAL #6/EVENING

9–11 P.M.   1 protein
            1 fruit
            8 ounces water

CARBOHYDRATE DAY
(WITH FIVE SUGGESTED FOOD CHOICES FOR EACH MEAL)

You should drink at least 8 ounces of water with all meals and snacks.

MEAL #1/WAKE UP (PREWORKOUT)

7–8 A.M.
1. 2 slices turkey bacon, 2 slices multigrain toast. Coffee (half caffeine/half decaf) or tea.

2. Cheese omelet: Mix together 1 egg and 1 slice low-fat cheddar or low-fat Swiss cheese. Pour into a nonstick skillet and heat through to prepare the omelet; 1 serving cooked oat bran cereal. Coffee (half caffeine/half decaf) or tea.

3. 1 serving oatmeal cooked with 2 tablespoons of chopped walnuts and ½ cup low-fat milk. Coffee (half caffeine/half decaf) or tea.

4. 2 hard-boiled eggs, 1 whole-wheat English muffin with 2 teaspoons natural peanut butter. Coffee (half caffeine/half decaf) or tea.

5. Bagel Breakfast Sandwich: Serve 2 scrambled egg whites between a sliced whole-wheat bagel. Coffee (half caffeine/half decaf) or tea.

WORKOUT

8–9 A.M.   8 ounces water

MEAL #2/POSTWORKOUT

9–10 A.M.
1. 1 whole-wheat English muffin, ½ cup unsweetened chunky-style applesauce.

2. 1 whole-wheat bagel, 1 pear.

3. 1 serving cooked multigrain cereal, ½ grapefruit.

4. 1 small bran muffin, 1 orange.

5. 1 cup oat bran, microwaved, with 1 cup sliced strawberries.

MEAL #3/LUNCH

12–1 P.M.
1. Tuna Pita Pocket: Mix tuna with 1 cup shredded lettuce, 2 tablespoons chopped tomato, 2 tablespoons chopped onion, and 1 tablespoon extra-virgin olive oil. Stuff into 1 piece of whole-wheat pita pocket bread.

2. Mini-Pizzas: Spread fat-free, sugar-free marinara sauce on both halves of a lightly toasted whole-wheat English muffin. Top with shredded low-fat mozzarella cheese and 2 tablespoons sliced mushrooms. Season to taste with Italian seasoning. Place under the broiler at medium heat until cheese melts. Serve with a tossed salad of salad

greens and salad veggies drizzled with 1 tablespoon extra-virgin olive oil and balsamic vinegar.

3. Grilled Chicken Caesar: Top 2 cups romaine lettuce with grilled chicken, slices of red onion, and 1 tablespoon grated Parmesan cheese. Drizzle with 1 tablespoon extra-virgin olive oil and balsamic vinegar and serve with whole-wheat crackers.

4. Egg Salad Sandwich: Chop two hard-boiled eggs and mix with 1 teaspoon yellow mustard, I teaspoon unsweetened relish, and 1 tablespoon extra-virgin olive oil. Spread egg mixture on 2 slices multigrain bread. Serve with baby carrots and chopped raw cauliflower.

5. Tofu Pasta: Mix together I serving tofu, ½ cup chopped zucchini, ½ cup chopped tomato, ½ cup chopped onion, and ½ cup sugar-free, fat-free marinara sauce. Heat until vegetables are soft. Serve over 1 cup whole-wheat pasta.

MEAL #4/MIDAFTERNOON

3–4 P.M.
1. Baked Apple: Bake apple in small baking dish with ¼ cup of water at 400 degrees until soft. Sprinkle with cinnamon and serve.

2. 1 cup chopped mango.

3. 1 cup blackberries.

4. ½ banana mixed with ½ cup sliced strawberries.

5. ½ of a honeydew melon.

MEAL #5/DINNER

6–7 P.M.
1. Broiled swordfish or mahimahi, ½ cup brown rice, steamed asparagus, and steamed yellow (summer) squash.

2. Eye of round steak; 3 small red potatoes, boiled; tossed salad with salad greens and salad veggies, drizzled with

THE BROWN FAT REVOLUTION EATING PLAN

1 tablespoon extra-virgin olive oil and 2 tablespoons red-wine vinegar.

3. Vegetarian Plate: Mix pinto beans or black beans with cooked brown rice, heat and top with 2 tablespoons of salsa; cooked corn, and steamed spinach.

4. Burger and Fries Dinner: Serve broiled lean ground turkey patty on a whole-wheat hamburger bun with lettuce, sliced tomato, and 1 tablespoon low-carb ketchup. Serve with Sweet Potato Fries: Cut 1 sweet potato in eighths, then slice each piece into strips like French fries. Place on a cookie sheet that has been sprayed lightly with vegetable cooking spray. Bake in a 400-degree oven for a half hour or until "fries" are cooked thoroughly.

5. Ahi tuna slices or grilled tuna steak, brown rice, steamed brussels sprouts, and steamed cauliflower. Serve with wasabi or low-sodium soy sauce for seasoning.

MEAL #6/EVENING

9–11 P.M.
1. 1 cup Greek-style yogurt, 2 sliced kiwifruits.

2. 1 serving tofu, 1 cup strawberries.

3. 1 handful almonds, 1 cup blueberries.

4. Peach Shake: Blend together 1 cup soy, low-fat, or skim milk with 1 cup frozen (unsweetened) peach slices.

5. Tuna mixed with ¼ mashed avocado.

EATING SCHEDULES IF YOU WORK OUT IN THE LATE AFTERNOON OR EVENING

PROTEIN DAY

MEAL #1/WAKE UP

7 A.M.
1 protein
1 carb
8 ounces water
1 cup coffee (half caffeine/half decaf) or tea

MEAL #2/MIDMORNING

9–10 A.M.
1 fruit
8 ounces water
Second cup of coffee (half caffeine/half decaf) or tea, if desired

MEAL #3/LUNCH

12–1 P.M.
1 protein
2 vegetables
8 ounces water

MEAL #4/MIDAFTERNOON (PREWORKOUT)

3–4 P.M.
1 fruit
8 ounces water

WORKOUT

5–6 P.M.
8 ounces water

MEAL #5/DINNER (POSTWORKOUT)

6–7 P.M.
1 protein
1 carb

2 vegetables

8 ounces water

MEAL #6/EVENING

10–11 P.M.   1 protein

1 fruit

8 ounces water

PROTEIN DAY

(WITH FIVE SUGGESTED FOOD CHOICES FOR EACH MEAL)

MEAL #1/WAKE UP

7 A.M.   1. Breakfast Quesadilla: Scramble 1 egg with 3 tablespoons shredded low-fat cheddar cheese, add to 1 corn tortilla, and top with 1 tablespoon salsa. Coffee (half caffeine/half decaf) or tea.

2. 2 scrambled eggs, 1 serving oatmeal. Coffee (half caffeine/half decaf) or tea.

3. Steak and eggs: 1 small portion grilled steak (2 to 3 ounces), 2 scrambled egg whites, 1 slice multigrain toast. Coffee (half caffeine/half decaf) or tea.

4. ½ cup low-fat cottage cheese sprinkled with 1 tablespoon chopped walnuts, 1 whole-grain bagel. Coffee (half caffeine/half decaf) or tea.

5. Cheesy Corn Grits: Cook grits according to package directions. Stir in 2 slices grated low-fat cheddar cheese and let melt. Add 1 tablespoon chopped jalapeño peppers, if desired. Coffee (half caffeine/half decaf) or tea.

MEAL #2/MIDMORNING

9–10 A.M.   1. 1 apple. Coffee (half caffeine/half decaf) or tea, if desired.

2. 1 cup watermelon cubes. Coffee (half caffeine/half decaf) or tea, if desired.

3. 2 peeled and sliced kiwifruits. Coffee (half caffeine/half decaf) or tea, if desired.

4. 1 cup sliced strawberries, with 4 teaspoons semisweet chocolate chips. Coffee (half caffeine/half decaf) or tea, if desired.

5. ½ grapefruit, sprinkled with cinnamon. Coffee (half caffeine/half decaf) or tea, if desired.

MEAL #3/LUNCH

12–1 P.M.

1. 3 slices white-meat turkey, 1 cup salad greens, and 1 cup chopped tomatoes, drizzled with 1 tablespoon extra-virgin olive oil with 2 tablespoons red-wine vinegar.

2. Tuna Lettuce Wraps: Combine tuna with 2 tablespoons chopped celery, 1 tablespoon fat-free mayonnaise, and 1 tablespoon unsweetened relish. Mix well and place in large iceberg lettuce leaves to form wraps. 1 cup baby carrots.

3. Chicken breast, grilled or baked; steamed spinach or other greens; and cooked carrots.

4. Chef Salad: Top a generous bed of salad greens with a hard-boiled egg, sliced in fourths, and 4 strips of low-fat cheese. Add other salad veggies as desired: grape tomatoes, chopped onions, chopped green pepper, etc. Toss with 1 tablespoon of extra-virgin olive oil and 2 tablespoons of balsamic vinegar.

5. Stuffed Tomato: Slice into a large tomato to create wedges, while still keeping the tomato intact. Fill the middle with ½ cup low-fat cottage cheese. Garnish the top with 1 tablespoon chopped pecans. Serve stuffed tomato on a generous bed of lettuce.

THE BROWN FAT REVOLUTION EATING PLAN

MEAL #4/MIDAFTERNOON (PREWORKOUT)

3–4 P.M.
1. 1 medium orange.

2. 1 banana.

3. Berry Mix: Combine ½ cup blueberries and ½ cup raspberries.

4. 1 apple.

5. 1 cup fresh cherries.

WORKOUT

5–6 P.M.   8 ounces water.

MEAL #5/DINNER (POSTWORKOUT)

6–7 P.M.
1. Grilled salmon or tuna steak, steamed zucchini, large tossed salad drizzled with 1 tablespoon extra-virgin olive oil and 2 tablespoons red-wine vinegar. ½ cup brown rice.*

2. Beef Stew: In a pan that has been lightly sprayed with vegetable spray, brown cubes of lean beef. Add in ¼ cup chopped onion, ¼ cup chopped green bell pepper, ½ cup sliced button mushrooms, and ½ cup tomato sauce. Season with ¼ teaspoon garlic powder and 2 teaspoons Worcestershire sauce. Cover saucepan and let simmer on low heat for 20 minutes. Serve with 1 medium whole-wheat dinner roll.*

3. 2 lean pork chops, steamed broccoli, steamed cauliflower, and ½ cup green peas.*

4. Baked turkey breast, steamed greens (spinach, kale, or turnip greens), steamed cauliflower, and ½ baked acorn squash.*

5. Baked white fish (any type), steamed asparagus, steamed yellow (summer) squash, and ½ cup brown rice.*

*On your nonworkout days, replace the carb with a nonstarchy vegetable of your choice.

10–11 P.M.

1. 1 cup Greek-style yogurt, mixed with ½ cup chunky unsweetened applesauce.

2. 2 slices low-fat cheese, 1 cup green or red grapes.

3. Peachy Shake: Blend together ½ cup nonfat peach-flavored yogurt, ½ cup low-fat milk, and 1 peeled and sliced peach.

4. 1 serving tofu, topped with 1 cup blueberries.

5. 1 cup low-fat or skim milk, 2 figs.

CARBOHYDRATE DAY

MEAL #1/WAKE UP

7 A.M.

1 protein
1 carb
8 ounces water
1 cup coffee (half caffeine/half decaf) or tea

MEAL #2/MIDMORNING

9–10 A.M.

1 fruit
1 cup coffee (half caffeine/half decaf) or tea, if desired.
8 ounces water

MEAL #3/LUNCH

12–1 P.M.

1 protein
1 carb
2 vegetables
8 ounces water

MEAL #4/MIDAFTERNOON (PREWORKOUT)

3–4 P.M.   1 carb
1 fruit
8 ounces water

WORKOUT

5–6 P.M.   8 ounces water

MEAL #5/DINNER (POSTWORKOUT)

6–7 P.M.   1 protein
1 carb
2 vegetables
8 ounces water

MEAL #6/EVENING

9–11 P.M.   1 protein, with or without fruit
8 ounces water

CARBOHYDRATE DAY
(WITH FIVE SUGGESTED FOOD CHOICES FOR EACH MEAL)

MEAL #1/WAKE UP

7 A.M.   1. ½ cup low-fat cottage cheese spread on 2 slices cinnamon-raisin toast. Coffee (half caffeine/half decaf) or tea.

2. 2 chicken sausage links, 2 slices whole-grain toast with 1 teaspoon butter. Coffee (half caffeine/half decaf) or tea.

3. 1 cup low-fat or skim milk, 1 cup high-fiber cereal (such as All-Bran, Bran Buds, or Fiber One). Coffee (half caffeine/half decaf) or tea.

4. Cheese Omelet: Whisk together 1 egg, 2 egg whites, and 1 tablespoon shredded low-fat cheese. Pour into a small

frying pan that has been sprayed lightly with vegetable spray. Cook over low to medium heat until cooked through. Fold and serve on a plate with 2 slices whole-grain toast. Coffee (half caffeine/half decaf) or tea.

5. 2 scrambled or poached eggs; 1 serving oatmeal topped with 1 tablespoon chopped walnuts, pecans, or almonds. Coffee (half caffeine/half decaf) or tea.

MEAL #2/MIDMORNING

9–10 A.M.

1. 1 banana, sliced and sprinkled with 1 tablespoon chopped walnuts. Coffee (half caffeine/half decaf) or tea, if desired.

2. Citrus Medley: Combine ½ cup chopped orange segments with ½ cup raspberries. Coffee (half caffeine/half decaf) or tea, if desired.

3. 1 pear. Coffee (half caffeine/half decaf) or tea, if desired.

4. ¼ wedge honeydew melon. Coffee (half caffeine/half decaf) or tea, if desired.

5. 1 nectarine. Coffee (half caffeine/half decaf) or tea, if desired.

MEAL #3/LUNCH

12–1 P.M.

1. Deli-Style Sandwich: Stack sliced roast beef, 1 slice reduced-fat mozzarella, lettuce, onion slices, and tomato slices on 2 slices whole-grain bread spread with 1 teaspoon yellow or dark mustard. 1 cup baby carrots.

2. 1 ground turkey patty, broiled on 1 whole-wheat hamburger bun with lettuce, onion slices, tomato slices. 1 cup chopped raw broccoli florets.

3. Salmon Salad: Place grilled salmon on generous bed of baby spinach leaves, ½ cup chopped cucumbers, and ½ cup chopped red or yellow bell pepper, drizzled with 1

tablespoon extra-virgin olive oil with 2 tablespoons red-wine vinegar. ½ cup brown rice.

4. Grilled chicken breast, 2 cups steamed mixed vegetables, ½ cup brown rice.

5. Grilled Cheese Sandwich: Place 2 slices low-fat American cheese between 2 slices whole-grain bread. Brown in a skillet that has been lightly sprayed with vegetable spray. Serve with sliced tomato and 1 cup baby carrots.

MEAL #4/MIDAFTERNOON (PREWORKOUT)

3–4 P.M.
1. 1 medium baked sweet potato, topped with ¼ cup chunky unsweetened applesauce.

2. 1 small bran muffin, 1 banana.

3. Whole-wheat crackers, 6 slices avocado.

4. 1 serving oatmeal or oat bran, microwaved with 1 diced peach.

5. Quick Trail Mix: Combine 1 cup high-fiber flaked cereal (such as bran flakes or Fiber One) with ¼ finely chopped dried apricot and 2 tablespoons chopped walnuts or almonds.

WORKOUT

5–6 P.M.   8 ounces water.

MEAL #5/DINNER (POSTWORKOUT)

6–7 P.M.
1. Beef Fajitas: Place slices of grilled flank steak, avocado slices, and salsa in two whole-wheat tortillas and fold over. Large tossed salad with assorted salad veggies drizzled with 1 tablespoon extra-virgin olive oil and 2 tablespoons red-wine vinegar.

2. Restaurant Dinner: grilled salmon, tossed salad with dressing on the side (oil and vinegar), vegetable medley, and ½ cup rice.

3. Steamed or boiled shrimp with cocktail sauce; steamed broccoli, cooked carrots, and ½ cup cooked corn or corn on the cob.

4. Chicken breast, grilled or baked; steamed green beans; steamed yellow (summer) squash; ½ cup cooked pearl barley or ½ cup whole-wheat pasta.

5. Pork tenderloin, medley of steamed zucchini and red bell peppers, 1 medium baked sweet potato.

MEAL #6/EVENING

9–11 P.M.

1. 2 slices low-fat cheddar cheese with optional pear.

2. 1 cup nonfat fruit-flavored yogurt with optional 1 cup of berries, any variety.

3. Fruit Parfait: Layer 1 cup Greek-style yogurt with 1 cup blueberries and 2 tablespoons sliced almonds in a parfait glass.

4. 1 cup low-fat or skim milk, optional 2 tangerines.

5. ½ cup low-fat cottage cheese mixed with optional ½ cup chunky unsweetened applesauce and a dash of cinnamon.

SUGGESTED SUPPLEMENTS TO HELP INCREASE FAT METABOLISM

Please refer to the list on page 114 in chapter 5.

PART III

THE BROWN FAT REVOLUTION EXERCISE PLAN

7.
HOW THE BROWN FAT REVOLUTION EXERCISE PLAN IS DIFFERENT

Do you remember those crazy, heady days of puberty, when your hormones kicked in and all of a sudden you didn't recognize your body anymore? When you had a lovely flat belly, soft rounded curves exactly where you wanted them, and firm, shapely breasts and arms?

And then, after many years of being comfortable with this body—the body that has given you pleasure in its strength and may have borne you children— you find yourself going through a sort of puberty in reverse when perimenopause and then menopause come along. Once again, your hormones are stirring, making changes to your mood and your appearance. Changes you basically have little control over. Changes that can often make you feel as if your body is betraying you.

These changes can be especially difficult to take if you've been diligent about regular exercise over the years. I've had patients (in their late thirties and up) who've spent countless hours in the gym, who took great pride in the fact that their hard work allowed them to be wearing the same dress size at forty that they wore at twenty, tell me that it's as if they woke up one morning and found that some stranger had suddenly appeared in their belly.

A stranger that's giving them the "middle-age spread" they thought would never happen to them.

A stranger, triggered by declining hormone levels, who appears in the form of soft and old yellow fat, making them soft and spongy instead of firm and lean.

"What's happening to me?" they ask. "I can't get rid of these ten pounds, no matter what I do. And they're all in my belly and my butt! You've got to help me!"

A STRONG CORE IS THE KEY

What is the goal of an exercise program? To maintain your physical health and give you strength, of course. But another important goal is to keep your body as youthful and vibrant as possible, no matter what your age.

I know that if you can't see truly visible results when you're on an eating or exercise regimen, it's almost impossible to want to continue on it no matter how "healthy" this regimen supposedly is. You need to see benefits to all your hard work and discipline.

So it is more than okay to want to push past the accepted and appropriate goal of better health, and say out loud: "I don't just want to be healthy—I want to look great, too!" Once you can do this, and once you start seeing the results of the Brown Fat Revolution, you'll be able to not only embrace the aging process but be perfectly calm in the face of it—because every time you look in the mirror you won't see a woman who's visibly growing older (and deteriorating as she does), but a woman who is firm and trim yet curvy in the right places, buoyed by her cushion of dense and resilient young brown fat.

What makes a woman's body look youthful is a strong core, or the center of your body from your shoulders down to your buttocks and thighs. Most of all, you want good brown fat in specifically targeted areas that define that youthfulness: your upper arms, hips, belly, buttocks, and, of course, your face.

This is what the Core Curriculum of my Exercise Plan will accomplish. The science behind it is based on the basic principle that you burn more fat if you increase your lean muscle—more than if you do long cardiovascular workouts. Cardio exercise increases your metabolism only *during* the workout, but building your lean muscle mass will raise your metabolic rate *around the clock*. And even though cardio exercise enlarges certain muscles, especially in your legs, don't forget you have dozens of muscles attached to the hips, pelvis, lower back, abdomen, ribs, and shoulders, too—your body's core.

Strengthening these core muscles is your most effective tool for raising your metabolism, and the best way to get rid of bad yellow fat.

Building lean muscle through the Core Curriculum increases your metabolism continuously for at least twenty-four hours after a workout; an intense cardio program only increases metabolism for several hours. And the benefits of the Core Curriculum go beyond weight control. You'll soon see changes in your body *shape*. The Core Curriculum will make your body lean, strong, more coordinated, and more shapely.

If you want real, long-term results, it's counterproductive to work out in the same way at fifty as you did when you were thirty-five. Since your female hormones (primarily estrogen and progesterone) define how, when, and where your body's fat distribution changes as you grow older, the Exercise Plan changes according to your age group. As with the Eating Plan, you'll be in either Hormone Category I (thirty to fifty) or Hormone Category II (fifty or older). In the following four chapters, you'll be given specific routines to do that will take the guesswork out of what areas to target and how to target them with maximum efficiency in minimal time.

In addition, the Exercise Plans for Hormone Category II are less intense and gentler to save your joints from potential stress and injury. They also emphasize exercises for specific areas of the body where changes are inevitable due to fat distribution, such as the lower abdomen and upper arms—areas that tend to be overlooked and underexercised.

Although spot reduction is not possible, with this Exercise Plan, contour changes in different parts of the body—especially in the problem areas associated with gender, age, and genetics—are managed by decreased overall yellow fat. This yellow fat, as you know, is loose and hanging since it's not firmly encased with connective tissue, leading to bulges and pooches. By diminishing the quantity of this fat in *all* areas of your body, your problem areas will improve and firm up, too.

And by focusing your workout in areas where yellow fat tends to be deposited, your muscles can be used to maintain firmness *below* the fat, such as in the lower abdomen. If you don't exercise and you do have a lot of yellow fat, picture your lower abdomen as having lax muscles and bulging internal organs, all topped with a thick layer of yellow fat. But once you start to flatten this layer with specific exercises, you'll see a real improvement. Couple this overall reduction in body fat with proper nutrition as well as a speedier metabolism thanks to increased lean muscle mass and a layer of firm, healthy brown fat, and your shape will change completely.

Having a trim, tight core is amazing—it's the "tummy tuck" of exercise. For this reason the exercises you'll be doing are specifically structured to strengthen the center of the body in three dimensions: top to bottom, side to side, and front to back. They add flexibility, stability, and balance; your core will support your spine so it's less prone to muscle strain, while also improving posture. Your overall strength will increase, too. These are all the essential elements of what you're looking for most—a *youthful* body.

THE GENESIS OF THE EXERCISE PLAN

I went from being a competitive ballroom dancer to an unfit and unhealthy Mallomar Man. I didn't exercise for twenty-two years. After finally admitting that if I didn't do something, I would be ruining my health (and potentially my career, because surgeons need to have stamina), I learned how to transform my body from flabby to lean, strong, shapely, and powerful. I became not just a bodybuilder, but a body sculptor. I literally transformed the entire shape of my body solely by using weights. I couldn't believe it. What I was capable of doing was fantastically empowering, on every possible level.

What I also realized, as I developed my program, was that any person who uses weights can feel the same way. Anyone can master the basic skills, no matter what their age, strength, or weight is when they start. It's not like an English speaker trying to learn a tonal-based language like Chinese at the age of forty-five, when acquiring that very specific set of mental and linguistic skills is difficult. Doing weight work is the great equalizer, done purely to improve your shape—and your health.

Think of this Exercise Plan as the physical complement to what you're already doing with the Eating Plan. The two together create a synergistic whole. While the Eating Plan will gradually change your body on the *inside*—transforming bad yellow fat into the kind of good brown fat that gives you firm curves—these exercises will reinforce the plan by keeping the surrounding muscles strong and toned, which will clearly be evident on the *outside*.

ABOUT THE CORE CURRICULUM

Most people erroneously believe that the core deals only with the muscles of the abdomen (or abs). Say "core" to them and they're going to immediately click into unpleasant thoughts of the endless crunches they've done over the years—crunches that probably never gave them the flat belly of their dreams.

THE CORE DEFINED

What is the core? It's actually the entire pillar, or center, of your body, starting from your shoulders down to your hips, the gluteus muscles of your buttocks (or glutes), and your thighs. It's a lot more than just your abdominal muscles.

All body strength comes from your core. The hunter/gatherers that we've evolved from used their cores every day, as they needed to be able to jump, twist, and crouch to be successful hunters and survive. Professional athletes use their core in order to be at the top of their game; take a look at how Venus and Serena Williams have transformed women's tennis because they understood the value of good weight training that centered around developing a strong and supple core, not just strong arms and shoulders and lightning-quick reflexes.

But most people are inactive, so they don't use their core muscles very much or very often. They sit down during work. They sit down while driving. They stay seated while eating and watching TV. And so their cores become soft and prone to injury and aches and pains, particularly their backs (which need support from core muscles).

Restoring and strengthening all the muscles of your core will give your body central stability and strength. A strong core is the foundation for a long, lean, and supple figure, with gorgeous straight posture and the shape of your youth.

The Core Curriculum works so well because it builds lean muscle mass, which increases your metabolism. Aerobic exercise has little effect on any bad yellow fat you may have surrounding your intestines, but a strong muscle wall can buttress the abdomen, leaving it taut and trim.

If you regularly do a sport or exercise that is dependent on a strong core—such as dancing, golf, or tennis—for the cardio component of your Exercise Plan, you'll not only automatically engage your core and reinforce your weight training, but have a lot of fun, too.

Since volume is all about fat, you also need to think of your core as being three-dimensional—more like a tube. It's not just about how you look from the front. You need to consider how you look in profile, and from the back, too. Which is why three-way mirrors in department-store changing rooms can be such an unpleasant shock.

If you were able to check your "tube" regularly, you'd be hyperaware that, thinking three-dimensionally, a weak core is extremely aging. It's the area of a woman's body that ages more quickly than anything else, especially if the woman has had children. But now you can set the clock back—once you embark on a dedicated program to firm up your core.

CORE WORK: ABDOMINALS

I've seen countless patients who tell me, "I do a thousand crunches, but look, I've still got a pooch. It's driving me crazy!"

Crunches alone aren't going to work on your pooch because they target only a few of the core muscles, not all the muscles that affect your three-dimensionality. As a very important part of the core, especially in women, all the abdominal muscles need to be toned and tightened—and they will be since the Core Curriculum targets all the muscles in the area.

Plus, as you lose your bad yellow fat thanks to the Eating Plan, the new strength you'll be developing in this area will become even more apparent.

Remember, in no other area of the body is the necessity to focus on diet and exercise more apparent than in the abdomen.

CORE WORK: BACK

Your lower back is part of your core, so whenever you work these muscles you'll automatically strengthen this area, which should lessen any back pain caused by muscle weakness. A strong back will also greatly improve your posture.

CORE WORK: BUTTOCKS/THIGHS—GLUTES, HAMSTRINGS, AND QUADS

When most trainers or exercise books talk about legs, they mean the entire leg from thighs on down to calves and ankles.

For this book, though, I want you to think of your legs in two parts, as we do medically when approaching surgical procedures. The area at the top part of your legs—the thighs (which includes the quadriceps, or quads, in the front and the hamstrings in the back) as well as the gluteus (glutes) group that makes up your buttocks—are considered as a whole when you do the exercises of the Core Curriculum. These are the biggest muscle groups that define core strength and tone.

CORE WORK: SHOULDERS

Once you have well-developed shoulder muscles, it's as if you have built-in designer shoulder pads. The shape and shadows of a rounded deltoid not only look beautiful, but the strong muscle group pulls the shoulder back in proper alignment with the pelvis, so that you no longer slouch and your breasts and arms look youthful.

Ideally, the shoulders and the abdomen should work together to create the posture of youth. Sure, you can exercise like crazy and have toned and defined muscles, but without proper alignment and good posture, they won't pop.

EXTREMITIES: ARMS AND CALVES

Your arms and your calves are worked out secondarily to your core.

As triceps start to sag, particularly with the Hormone Category II group, it's especially important to concentrate on strengthening the arm.

The leg workout will prime and develop your calves, giving you a beautiful diamond-shaped pair of muscles (the gastrocnemius and soleus) that balances your thigh muscles (and also makes you look great in high heels!).

TAILORING THE CORE CURRICULUM

HORMONE CATEGORY I

In your thirties, your fat is starting to shift to your hips and thighs. These exercises will build a strong core, increase lean muscle, and include sprints for cardiac health, respiratory reserve, and maximal efficiency of exercise.

Because this is the decade when many women have children, exercises will also focus on restoring muscle tone to the abdomen after pregnancy.

In your forties, your fat is starting to move slightly toward the upper arms, but you're more likely to be seeing changes in your buttocks, hips, and thighs. You can also continue the sprint cardio exercises to increase metabolism and burn fat, and add intermittent circuit training.

HORMONE CATEGORY II

As you approach menopause and beyond, hormonal diminishment means that fat redistribution is inevitable, especially to your abdomen, buttocks, breasts, arms, and in other areas, too. Your overall body shape will tend to thicken, giving you less of an hourglass figure.

These are the decades where regular exercise is the *most* important. You'll continue with your Core Curriculum to maintain a flexible, slender waist, improved posture and balance, and increased stamina.

CORE CURRICULUM BASICS

DIFFERENT CORE ROUTINES

There are several core routines, but you perform only a few per day, and not every day. These routines are covered in chapters 9–12.

For those at the Beginner/Intermediate level as well as the Intermediate/Advanced level, the exercise routines should take no more than thirty minutes.

Depending on whether you're in Hormone Category I or Hormone Category II, the routines will alternate in different patterns of Core Days (I, II, and III), Extremities Day, Cardio Day, and Off Day.

On different Core Days, you'll be given exercises from these categories: Abdomen and Shoulders, Glutes and Hamstrings, and Quads and Lower Back.

On Extremities Day, you'll work your arms (biceps and triceps) and calves (gastrocnemius and soleus).

Hormone Category II will have an additional Abdomen/Triceps Day, targeting the areas of the body that need extra work as you grow older.

On Cardio Days, you can do whatever physical activity you like—dancing, swimming, tennis, racquetball, a brisk walk, etc.—but if you choose to get on a machine (such as a treadmill, elliptical, rower, or stair-stepper) at the gym (what is usually thought of as "cardio"), do *no more* than thirty minutes total, and try to do sprinting because it's extremely efficient. (I never do more than twenty minutes of sprinting-type cardio, ever! See page 148 for more on the Sprinting Method.)

Obviously, there's no question that cardiovascular exercise is good for your heart, lungs, and circulation. But as you know, I want you to move away from the concept of cardio as the primary way to control your weight or to develop your core muscles. It just can't do that for you.

And Off Day means don't work out! Your muscles truly need the rest in order to replenish themselves.

WORK ALL YOUR CORE MUSCLES

No one has a perfectly symmetric body, where all areas react the same way to exercise. Some women see their arms become beautifully buff in only a few weeks while their butts don't seem to change at all in the same time period. Or vice versa.

What I see in the gym every time I go is that people have favorite parts of their bodies and they keep working on them because it makes them feel good. And then they'll feel good that they exercised, but they haven't really exercised *properly*. Or they'll get tired and forget to do the rest of their exercises so they have a balanced routine that helps all muscle groups.

For instance, I used to see a guy in my gym with the biggest arms I've ever seen. They were humongous. Every day he did his arms—and nothing else. He just loved their shape so much he forgot about the rest of his body.

Don't fall into the same trap he did. You need to find the determination to attack the weakest area of your body, too. (You might even want to work it first, to get it out of the way.)

THESE EXERCISES ARE EASY TO DO

These exercises are all simple enough to do on your own, with *only* a bungee cord as your primary piece of equipment, so you don't need a trainer. Nor do you need to do any of these exercises in a gym—you can do them all at home, or on the road in your hotel room, or at a friend's when you're traveling. If you want to hire a trainer to jump-start your workout program and help you learn the routines, that's fine. But I do hope that eventually you'll be self-motivated enough and enjoy the routines so much that you'll be able to work out on your own.

THESE EXERCISE ROUTINES ARE QUICK

Your routines should take no longer than thirty minutes, no matter what your level. As you already know, more time spent doing hard-core cardio can be counterproductive, not only to the body but especially to the face. But if you want to ramp it up, cardio should be done at the end of the workout and for no more than fifteen minutes (bringing your total time to forty-five minutes).

As for when you do your Core Curriculum exercises, the morning is optimal—morning exercise will charge your metabolism and clear your mind for the day—but many people prefer evening workouts. The most important thing is that you make time for exercise.

CUT DOWN ON CARDIO—THE OVEREXERCISING PARADOX

One of the biggest differences between my exercise philosophy and that of most other exercise plans is that I consider aerobic exercise as secondary to the Core Curriculum, *not* the primary exercise. But you might be surprised at how short and how moderate these cardio workouts can be, and still be good for you. Also, while cardio is great for your heart and lungs, it can't build you the shape and contour of a youthful body, or replace your yellow fat with brown fat, either.

Lots of my patients suffer from Overexercise Syndrome—they've come to believe that cardio is almost infinitely beneficial and can't be overdone. But it can.

The skinny overexerciser doesn't eat before or after exercise, depleting her stores of glycogen and fat, so her starved body starts to digest muscle for energy. As a result, she might be thin, but her muscles are slack and her skin is wrinkled; still, her mind keeps encouraging her to continue working out for fear of gaining weight (which is precisely what she *needs* to do).

ABOUT THE SPRINTING METHOD

The best cardio for maximum benefits in minimal time is an activity that works out several muscle groups at once. If you choose to work out in a gym, my recommendations would be to use the stationary bike, stair-stepper, treadmill, or elliptical machine, or to go swimming.

Whatever cardio you choose, be sure it's an activity you truly enjoy: a bike ride, a stint on the stair-stepper, or something as simple as a brisk walk. It could be boxing with a sparring partner, senior swim with friends, or ballroom dancing, which worked for me. Or tennis or golf, which are often as much fun socially as they are good for your body. You can even join an adult team at your local YMCA or school, as much for the camaraderie as for the sport.

Still, it's not so much what you do for cardio, but *how* you do it. In my opinion, the Sprinting Method is the most efficient form of cardio if you want to have a great-looking body, maintain healthy brown fat, and get a superior heart-thumping exercise. (This is not sprinting, as in running a fast race, but my version of interval training.)

With the Sprinting Method, you do a movement as fast and hard as you can physically do it until you just can't continue any longer, at which point you slow back down while doing the same movement, lowering your heart rate. As soon as you feel the urge and ability, you then pump it up again as fast and hard as you can. You'll repeat this sequence as much as possible; obviously, how well you can sprint at first is based on how fit and how used to doing this kind of exercise you are.

Doing twenty minutes of Sprinting Method cardio is more than enough to burn yellow fat, get your heart going and your lungs working, and stimulate lean muscle development. Innumerable studies have shown that high intensity/short duration exercise like sprinting burns many more calories than long, low intensity exercise like jogging or walking. In addition, sprinting increases growth hormone, which enhances the immune system, promotes fat redistribution (away from the abdomen!), and increases lean muscle mass in addition to signaling fast-twitch fibers in muscle. (These are the fibers that grow in response to exercise.)

In my opinion, sprinting is the most efficient form of cardio as well as the best way to lose fat and gain muscle. If you're interested in getting a great-looking body, maintaining healthy brown fat, and getting a superior heart-thumping exercise, you might want to consider it.

I also find sprinting to be much more invigorating and much less boring than long sessions of lower-intensity cardio. It might work for you, too.

The overweight overexerciser does lose fat once she depletes her glycogen stores, but she will tend to overeat in response to overexercising, and the excess calories will automatically be stored as fat.

These overexercisers need to understand that too much exercise will lead you to a plateau where you stop improving. The reason is that cardio breaks everything down, so that even though you're increasing your metabolism during your workout and for several hours afterward, as well as getting rid of some fat and burning some calories, you're also stressing your muscles. Your body goes into complete starvation mode, holding on to every pound for survival.

The Brown Fat Revolution is designed to optimize muscle function, prevent joint strain, and build volume in areas that define beauty and youth. In order for muscles to properly grow, they must have a recovery period after every workout. It is the repair and replenishment of the muscle and the new growth that follows that adds a noticeable difference in muscle volume. Science has shown that the optimal period for muscle repair, when they need nutrients, water, and carbohydrates, is forty-eight hours for small muscles (like biceps and calves) and seventy-two hours for larger muscles (like glutes, hamstrings, and back).

WHAT ABOUT MY CARDIO ENDORPHIN RUSH?

Using your muscles often triggers a release of endorphins, which are compounds produced by the hypothalamus and the pituitary gland in your brain during excitement, exercise, orgasm, and pain; they give a sense of well-being during pleasurable activities. As endorphins flood your body, they can help you keep moving, thrilled to the potent power of your own wonderful body—which is why they're commonly referred to as a "runner's high."

But it's a fallacy to believe that doing a cardio workout is the only way to get an endorphin release. Anyone who does some form of regular exercise, such as that in the Brown Fat Revolution plan, or yoga, or Pilates, for example, can be flooded with endorphins, too—often much more easily and quickly than they would be during their old cardio routines.

If you don't give your muscles time to replenish themselves, eventually you'll go from productive exercise to *destructive* exercise. Sure, doing too much cardio might get rid of your yellow fat, but then it will get rid of all your brown fat and healthy muscle tissue, too. You'll think you're getting stronger while you're actually putting your body under attack. Your muscles will be unable to grow if they don't get any rest. You'll look gaunt, particularly in your face. You'll have less energy. Your breasts and arms will shrink. Your core might appear thin, but it won't be defined and firm (because there's no dense brown fat in it). You'll also be much more prone to injuries, and will take longer than usual to heal because your muscles and fat stores have been so depleted; then you'll obsess about not exercising and starve yourself so you won't gain weight, which will further send your body into starvation mode, and the vicious cycle of yo-yo dieting will begin.

As soon as overexercisers cut down on cardio and concentrate on their core instead—as well as change their eating habits to eat carbs before and after their workouts—their bodies will be transformed. Ideally, you should use the cardio element of your workout to keep your heart and lungs strong and your circulation flowing. But don't do what many women do, which is get upset after putting on a few pounds, run off to the gym, do an hour and a half of cardio, overdo it, and feel awful and too sore to keep on exercising. If these women had only done ten minutes of cardio and twenty minutes of weight training, they would not have felt so crummy.

Please don't think of cardio as the controller of your fat—because it isn't! Use it for fun, health benefits, or stress reduction, but only in moderation.

EQUIPMENT YOU'LL NEED

The equipment you'll need is minimal. See page 159 in chapter 8.

STICKING TO THE SCHEDULE

The workout schedule of Core Days, Extremities Day, Abdomen/Triceps Day for Hormone Category II, Cardio Day, and Off Days has been designed for optimal results, giving your muscles the proper balance of getting worked with time off.

While you need to stick to the program and do all the exercises in each section, you can certainly change the *order* you do them in. Feel free to mix it all up, although I have already worked this "mix-up" into your monthly workout schedule.

One of the signs of a poor exercise trainer is that he or she has the client do the same thing every time. That's counterproductive, because your body quickly accommodates itself to exercise, and then it can't improve unless you challenge it. Muscles respond to work—and they're not really getting worked unless you feel it. That's the classic "burn"—which should never be painful, but which should make you aware that the muscle is doing what you want it to. You won't feel this burn unless you challenge it and mix it up.

Even though I've been bodybuilding for decades, I still vary my routine every single time I work out—whether with the exercises themselves, the order of exercises, the repetitions, the amount of the weights, you name it, as you'll see in the next chapter.

WHAT ABOUT STRETCHING?

Although the many studies I've read have salient points about whether or not stretching pre- or postexercise helps your muscles work most efficiently, I believe in stretching *before* a workout. With the Core Curriculum, you will stretch the muscles of the day, bringing blood supply to those muscles and lubricating your joints before you start.

By stretching the muscle before working it out, you're doing what I call cognitive prep for the workout— you're sending a signal to your brain that you're about to get going on your circuit. As a result, your workout will be much more focused and effective.

That said, there are plenty of days when I'm not really in the mood to push it. On those days, I do a light workout. I listen to my body and what it's telling me it needs. But even if I'm tired or stressed or crabby, I still do my workout.

Whatever your mood or energy level, the most important thing is to try not to miss a session. As soon as you start, the endorphins should kick in and your stress should melt away, making you feel a whole lot better as your muscles get stronger.

You might not believe you're capable of any of this when you first start. But your growth will be exponential. You might take a bit of time to get going as you master the basics, but then suddenly you'll *get* it—and you'll start to fly.

MOVING ON TO THE NEXT LEVEL

As you'll see in chapters 10 and 12, there are detailed workouts for those who have mastered the Beginner/Intermediate level and are ready for a more intense session.

But instead of making you confused with an entirely different set of exercises, I'm going to combine the basics in unique ways—so you'll be able to master them more quickly and see faster results. Who can remember how to do twenty different biceps exercises? Not me! But you can easily remember four or five exercises per muscle group, and then be able to add some variations. And once you're more confident with your form, and using weights or the bungee cord has become second nature to you (which happens *very* quickly, believe it or not), you can really have fun during your workout.

This deliberate mix-up is not only fun, but the more muscle "confusion" you can introduce in a short span of time, the more your muscles need to work. That's because muscles quickly adapt to how they're used. If you do the same exercise over and over again, your muscle will not be stimulated and you'll have unproductive workouts. So one of the basic principles of body contouring is to change routines frequently so that muscles do not accommodate and get lazy. Modifying the type of exercise, number of reps, and sequence of reps should give you optimal results in extremely efficient workouts.

BEFORE YOU START:
DO A SELF-ASSESSMENT OF YOUR BODY

Now that you know the basics of how the Core Curriculum works, you still need a little bit of preparation before you get going.

The best way to do this is with a simple yet tough-to-do self-assessment, where you stand in front of a mirror, by yourself (and with no interruptions), and take a good, hard, honest look at your body.

Start at the top and move down. Assess your good and bad. What parts of your body are the strongest? What looks best when you're standing? What looks best when you're sitting? What looks best in profile?

A self-assessment will help your realize that your body has a certain shape and contour that is uniquely yours. Some of these elements are entirely out of your control, such as your height, your body shape, the size of your bones, and the size and shape of your features.

The other elements, such as your weight and the strength of your muscles, are entirely within your control. And if you truly want to form a shape and contour that's going to make you look strong, lean, and younger, you need to be specific. So if, for example, you've already got nice strong arms with firm, jiggle-free triceps, you don't have to do extra arm exercises, even if you love them. Keep your arms in shape with maintenance exercises and move on to other areas you might have ignored.

Being able to pinpoint areas you like and areas you don't will help you zone in on your program. And you'll have a much deeper satisfaction when you finally get rid of the pooch that's driven you crazy for twenty years!

SHOULD I MEASURE MYSELF BEFORE I START?

One of the reasons it's so important to do a self-assessment before you start is that it truly is amazing to stand in front of a mirror on a regular basis and see the results of your transformation. If you ever need a jolt to help you stick to the program, visible results can do the trick, especially if they are for parts of the body that might not ever have been toned and trim before.

Measuring yourself before you start the program is a decision only you can make. Measurement implies change in size, not pounds; when you tone your muscles, you're not necessarily losing weight—you're gaining the right kind of firm weight while increasing your metabolism and getting rid of blobby weight. This plan isn't about bulk—it's about lean.

Personally, I like measurements, especially once I see the numbers moving—

but I also know that it's more important to see the changes when you look in the mirror, and feel the changes when you put on your clothes. So if you're not sure if you want to measure or not, you might want to measure only your waist, as you should notice remarkable changes there. And try on your tightest jeans before you begin and then try them on a month later. If you've stuck to the program, I guarantee that you'll see a dramatic change in the way your jeans fit at the waist and in the thighs. They'll be a lot roomier.

This will also work with a sleeveless shirt, especially if you've been working hard on your arms. Seeing them look "cut" can be a magical moment for women who've hidden their arms for years out of embarrassment.

GETTING YOURSELF MOTIVATED

You can get anything you want in life. I really believe that anything is possible. Unless you're suffering from an injury or illness, your body can do almost anything you want it to do, in ways you once might have thought unimaginable.

You just have to make the decision to go there. It may take you a year; it may take you twenty years, but when you reach your goal, the pleasure you'll take in your success will be sweet indeed.

Getting motivated and staying motivated is as much of an emotional workout as doing exercises is a physical workout. You can't have one without the other.

This is because your body is unique to you, and your goals are unique to you, and your self-judgment is unique to you. But it can be very difficult to believe how unique you really are, something I've discussed at length with my self-conscious patients over the years.

The first hump you have to get over is tackling the little voice in your head from gym class. You know, the

USE VISUALIZATION TO HELP YOU REACH YOUR GOALS

Visualizing when you train can be incredibly helpful. Imagine how strong and buff and toned your upper arms will be after a few months of weight training.

Another trick is to put a wish picture on your refrigerator or in your home as a reminder to stay on course. Professional athletes are taught to see themselves on the podium receiving their medals after they demonstrate their nearly superhuman prowess, and this same method can work with everything in life. So whenever my abs need an extra bit of work, I put a photograph of a model with an amazing six-pack up on the mirror in my bathroom. Even after all this time exercising, I still need cues to help me visualize my goals.

Surround yourself with inspiration, whether visual, musical, intellectual, or spiritual, and you will always find yourself rising to levels that you never imagined for yourself.

one that says: "You can't do it, you're a klutz, you're no good, you're ugly, you're fat." In order to work out most effectively—and to take pleasure in your accomplishments—you need to banish all negativity, including that little voice telling you you're fat (when you aren't) or clumsy (when you aren't) or that you don't deserve to have a youthful figure again (when you do).

The second hump to get over is to not get discouraged when friends or loved ones are critical of what you're trying to accomplish.

It might sound corny, but at the end of the day, you've got to push past those humps. Just as you can learn to embrace the notion that fat is your friend, you can learn to love your body, too.

FINDING THE TIME TO EXERCISE

The questions I always ask my patients when they tell me they don't have the time to exercise are: "If you could do something in only a very short amount of time that is guaranteed to make you feel good, why won't you do it? Why do you want to feel bad and look bad?"

Frankly, if President Obama can find the time to work out several times a week, you can, too. He's a brilliant example, as was President Bush, of people who have great responsibilities and not enough hours in the day to tend to all of them, yet who have their priorities in order when it comes to staying fit. They know that regular exercise helps you work more efficiently, sleep more soundly, be healthier, manage stress, and have some much-needed time to yourself.

Simply put—make the time. Anyone can find thirty minutes during the day to work out, especially as you don't need to work out every day on the Brown Fat Revolution program. If you work in an office, you can shut the door and do your routine at lunchtime, as you won't be sweating very much during the weight-training portion of your workout.

A workout buddy can also be a great motivator. One of the reasons exercise classes and Weight Watchers are so successful is as much because of the camaraderie they offer as the work they put you through. If you schedule workouts (as well as your Eating Plan) with a friend, you're less likely to cancel, and you can track each other's progress and give each other motivation and support. Workout buddies are also great for the cardio component of your exercise routine; it can be a lot of fun to sweat with a friend!

You don't even need to be in the same place to work out together—you can both set a time to do your sessions and check in with each other before and after.

BALANCE IS EVERYTHING

Surgeons are trained to think with a certain dispassion—to have the ability to turn off all external stimuli in order to be able to focus on a life-threatening scenario. But doctors need to be able to turn off that dispassion when they deal with their personal lives, or they'll find themselves emotionally unbalanced.

I'm bringing this up because it relates not only to emotional balance (especially being there for your loved ones) but also to physical balance. You need both in order to be healthy.

Without that component of balance in your life, you'll burn out. Nothing will run as smoothly as it could if you prioritized what's really important. It took me decades before I realized how important it is to have movement be a daily part of my life. Don't miss out on decades of good health and looking your best, like I did. It's never too late to make the kind of changes that are all about improving yourself.

This is your journey. Don't let anyone push you off the road.

YOU'RE NEVER TOO OLD

Not long ago, an older woman came in to see if she might be a suitable candidate for a face-lift—at the tender age of seventy-three. I told her she was an absolute inspiration to me, and that every one of my patients who was bummed out about turning fifty, thinking that life was over, ought to have a word with her.

"Oh, heck, honey," she said, giving me a casual wave and a smile, "I'm not ready to go quite yet. My mother lived to be ninety-five, and my father lived to be ninety-eight. One day, when my mother was ninety-three and we were in Palm Beach, we wanted to go swimming. She went to the diving board and did a perfect swan dive, and then she got out of the pool, walked over to me, and asked, 'Were my toes pointed?'"

This woman and her fabulous mother both realized that their bodies were a tremendous source of fun and pleasure. Finding a physical activity you love is the key to a lifetime of using your body to balance your mind; otherwise, the daily stress of your busy life will drain all of your energy, making you look and feel old. Ballroom dancing, tap-dancing, swimming, hiking, bicycling, rowing, belly dancing, tennis, walking—these are the kinds of physical activities that should make you feel good, and feel happy, for a lifetime.

FIND WAYS TO BRING MORE HAPPINESS INTO YOUR LIFE, TOO

All the work on your health will be undermined if you don't find ways to cut the emotional fat from your life, and concentrate on happiness and positive thinking.

Finding the time to do something you truly love and that makes you happy—and making that an active part of your life—will always make you feel stronger and more confident. It will also help you manage the stresses that beset all of us.

And if you don't like doing something (as long as it's not part of your must-do list, like the commute to your job, or folding the laundry), then don't do it! I was reminded of how many people keep on doing things they don't like when I was talking to a friend of my wife's recently. This woman is an avid reader, and she was complaining about the book she'd just gotten out of the library. I asked her why she'd finished it if she disliked it so much, and she told me she felt *obligated*.

I have to say, I was a bit astonished. Why waste time on a library book you find yourself loathing just to say "I finished it"? Why run on a treadmill if it doesn't feel great? Why go to an exercise class where the teacher snubs you? Why eat carrots if you're not crazy about them?

If you made a choice to do something and then you discover that it doesn't connect to you in a truly positive way, cut your losses and move on. In fact, you're likely to stop anyway, which is fine—just as long as you don't let that bad experience dissuade you from starting again with something else you might like a whole lot more. Some-

---

LET THE MUSIC MOVE YOU

I've been training for twenty years, and even I need a kick in the rear sometimes. Meaning that I can get a little bit lazy and automatically click into autopilot—because it's easier to do that than to challenge myself.

One year, when I knew I had to crank it up a notch after my holiday eating got the better of my belly, I smartly updated my iPod. Hearing all new music instantly made me feel inspired, and I found it much easier to mix it up during my workout session because the music got me going.

Music will always make a workout seem quicker and easier. If you use an iPod or MP3 player, you can create a playlist that's timed to the speed of your workout. When you're starting out slow you want a certain beat; in the middle of your workout, when either you're starting to drag or you're needing to do a particular exercise that you've never been crazy about, put on your favorite song that makes you happy. It will make the time go much faster, and it will rev up your heart so you'll work harder without thinking about it.

When I do my weight training, I find myself doing my reps in tune with the music. By changing up the rhythm, I'm changing up the routine. When I use songs with different beats, I'm constantly challenging my muscles as I adjust my own speed to the rhythmic beat.

thing that will give you more endorphins, and will keep you in the game because you're stoked about what you're doing.

And I'm not just talking about exercise, but about everything important in life—good food, good relationships, good job, good communication, and a good and happy home. If any of these are skewed, everything else can tumble down like a house of cards built on a slippery table.

There are countless different ways that you can find something you love and that makes you happy. It can be learning a new hobby, going back to an old hobby, or going back to school. Nor need it be something you have to do on your own. As with having a workout buddy, sharing a goal, new skill, or pursuit with a friend or loved one will not only motivate you more, but will keep you at it and give you a camaraderie that will provide countless hours of pleasure.

What's the worst that can happen if you try? You might realize you're not as crazy about doing something as you thought you would be. If so, move on and find something else. Set the notch a little bit higher up or turn it in a different direction completely to tweak yourself out of your daily routine. After all, what passionate, intelligent woman wants to follow the same routine for her entire life? Aren't we lucky that we live in a world where constant reinvention is a real possibility?

Be like the ninety-three-year-old woman who loved to dive. Get out there and dive in yourself.

A FINAL WORD ABOUT EXERCISE: START SMALL, AND BELIEVE IN YOURSELF

The Brown Fat Revolution is not about making drastic changes that might have immediate results for a few weeks or months and then leave you feeling and looking worse than you did before. If you start small, beginning by taking baby steps, then you can't fail. You will always learn to walk, in however much time is necessary for you to learn how to stand up and move by yourself. This plan is about making profound changes—changes that will *last*—not cosmetic changes.

But when you're just starting a program, just learning the new language of how to eat and how to move, and you haven't quite mastered the lingo or seen any drastic differences in your clothing yet, it can be hard to believe that six months down the line you will have lost your craving for sugar, or that you will have beautifully toned upper arms and a smooth, trim belly and butt; youthful contours back in your face; and more energy than you dreamed possible.

The longer you stay on this program, the more your confidence will blossom even as your yellow fat melts away. And you will have the immense self-satisfaction of knowing that you set these goals, you achieved these goals, and you did it all by yourself.

So I'm all for you finding whatever it takes to keep you motivated and improve your performance. You deserve to reward yourself with your own time—time devoted to your body. Rushing through your workout to get back to the demands of the day is as counterproductive as doing the exercises with the wrong form. You won't see results as quickly as you would if you wholeheartedly dedicated that thirty minutes to you. Surely you deserve at least that much time to yourself every day!

Furthermore, when you work out effectively you're going to eat effectively, because the last thing you'll want to do is undo all your own hard work. But if you aren't prepared to do the things (like eating well and working out well) that will make you feel good and look good, you'll have a much tougher time sticking to this or any other program.

So start small. Stay positive. You are capable of much more than you ever believed possible.

The Brown Fat Revolution is not a race. It's not a comparison study to the diets or weight loss of your friends or loved ones. It's a program for life—*your* life.

8.
EXERCISE HOW-TO'S

BEFORE YOU START

EQUIPMENT YOU'LL NEED

The first and most important piece of equipment you'll need is an exercise bungee cord, also called an elastic resistance cord or exercise band. (You'll need two.) These come in different tension levels that are color-coded to show increasing levels of resistance, from yellow (easiest) to green, blue, red, and black (hardest). They are easily purchased online, are inexpensive, and are easy to transport and store.

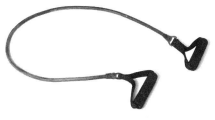

bungee cord

Since women do not want to bulk up when they work out, the Core Curriculum is designed to help them become trim and toned; to tighten, lift, and strengthen the core; and to contour and strengthen extremities—all with the use of a simple bungee cord. By using the bungee for resistance, both the positive (contraction) and the negative (relaxation) phases of muscle movement are simultaneously worked. Several studies have documented that these exercise bands are the most efficient way to achieve long, lean, and cut muscles. This is a much better result than the enormously thick muscles preferred by bodybuilders, who use heavy weights to stimulate the large fibers in their muscles, which creates bulk.

You should buy at least two levels of resistance, since different areas of your body, such as your arms and legs, will always have variable levels of muscle strength. You also may find that you rapidly progress and can handle greater resistance.

You will also need the following:

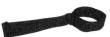

**door anchor
strap**

- Door anchor strap. This can be purchased online with the bungee cord.

- Two three-inch metal clasps for the bungee cord. These are also sold online. Some bungee sets allow you to attach ankle straps or different handles

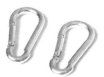

metal clasps

to the cord by securing it with a metal clasp. (Most bungee cords have a plastic handle at each end.)

- Padded ankle strap. This wraps around your ankle so you can attach the bungee cord to it, and is used for resistance movements as you take your leg through exercises toward the front (quads), toward the posterior or back (glutes and hamstrings), to the side in an outward direction (abductors), and across your body sideways (adductors).

padded ankle strap

- Exercise mat or comfortable, nonskid rug.

- Two solid, armless chairs.

- Optional: Exercise bench.

- Optional: Hand weights (two each) in two, five, or eight pounds, for experienced exercisers.

ABOUT THE EXERCISES

I am always amazed when I see the number of different exercises that are proposed in fitness magazines. To me, exercise is very straightforward. What's much more important than a huge variety of exercises is how you do a few good ones. The greater the number of exercises you do, the more likely you are to get confused and make mistakes in form, which will undermine the results of all your hard work. I see women in the gym every day, reading exercise directions out of little notebooks. They look perplexed and frustrated. And they really don't have to be.

The Brown Fat Revolution exercises are all tried-and-true basics that have shaped and strengthened me and my patients for over twenty years. They are simple to do, and they will give you maximum results with minimal stress on your joints.

Because you will get the best results when you focus on the quality and quantity of a few key movements, I have intentionally structured a program that will easily become familiar to you. These exercises will allow you to control the muscles of your body, and actually feel them contracting and toning.

You will also note that the difference between Beginner/Intermediate and Intermediate/Advanced is not the number of exercises but how they are done. You'll be adding on as dancers do; first by mastering the basic steps and then by adding on different variations into unique sequences.

MAKING YOUR WEIGHT TRAINING MORE EFFECTIVE

- Pay attention to your form. Focus on the quality of the movement as well as your position, balance, and control.

- Breathing is important: Keep it deliberate, relaxed, steady, and slow.

- Don't "swing" the weight back and forth.

- Take no more than one minute to rest between sets.

- When using the bungee cords, start with a yellow one, which has the lowest resistance. Move up gradually.

- Use a bungee cord (or the optional hand weights) with a resistance strength that causes your muscles to fatigue, or to feel the burn, at eight repetitions. (Taking a muscle to fatigue is good, as it's how a muscle grows and shapes itself.) *Never* move up to higher resistance with the bungee (or the weights) until you are completely comfortable with all movements and the number of repetitions.

  If you do choose to use hand weights, follow these guidelines:

  – Absolute beginners should start at no more than 1–2 pounds in each hand.

  – Beginners use 2–3 pounds.

  – Intermediate exercisers use 3–5 pounds.

  – Intermediate/advanced exercisers use 5–8 pounds.

  – Advanced exercisers use 8–10 pounds.

- Visualize a perfect shape to the body part that you are exercising.

- When the exercise is in full contraction, perform a deliberate contraction before slowly releasing.

- Mix it up to get the best results; muscles are incredibly adept at adapting to exercises.

- Eat preexercise meals that are easily digestible and not heavy on calories or fat—and that contain carbohydrates, since your body requires them to build lean muscle mass.

YOUR WORKOUT SCHEDULE

As explained earlier, your core consists of the abdomen, shoulders, glutes, hamstrings, quads, and lower back. The schedule you'll follow will strengthen them and give them the rest time they need.

It's human nature to want changes in some areas more than others, so you might be prone to subconsciously sabotaging the parts that are more difficult to work on and/or overworking the areas of the body that really bother you (such as by doing a ton of abs work and neglecting the upper body). This workout schedule is specifically designed for total body balance, which is the key to getting the shape you truly want.

These routines should take no more than thirty minutes.

The amount of repetitions (reps)/sets should be ten reps in three sets, with a minute's rest in between. Sometimes, though, you might not be able to get each set to ten reps, and that is okay. Work only to your limit, or when you feel the burn.

WHAT IF I MISS A DAY?

Even with the best intentions, life gets in the way. No one can always stick to the schedule, as much as you might want to.

If you miss a day, simply pick up where you left off. Do not skip that body part.

If you know in advance that you need to be off on a day within the sequence, feel free to place it anywhere in the cycle without any loss of muscle momentum. Off Days and Cardio Days can be interspersed anywhere. For example, you could change the schedule from what's listed here to Core I, Off, Extremities, Core II, Cardio, Off, Core III. Then start again with Core I. It's more important to do the Core and Extremities Days than the Cardio Day.

Make sure you have two days off each week!

MOVING ON TO THE NEXT LEVEL: FOR THOSE WHO ARE INTERMEDIATE/ADVANCED

What differentiates a beginner from an experienced exerciser is not the ability to perform a lot of different exercises, but the ability to do a few exercises perfectly, with the correct form and range of motion. So you should not consider doing any work at the Intermediate/Advanced level until you have completely mastered all the exercises in chapter 9, and you are comfortable doing them with perfect form.

In chapters 10 and 12 (Intermediate/Advanced), you'll see the same exercises as in chapters 9 and 11 (Beginner/Intermediate), but tweaked with elements from the following list to make them more challenging. Trust me, these maneuvers will all produce a "burn" even for the most advanced and experienced athletes! I've been doing these exercises for twenty years, so I know these movements really do work. The big difference here is how you'll be adjusting these exercises to keep the workouts fresh and even more potent.

You will notice that not every exercise has suggested add-ons to mix it up. This is deliberate, because even at the Intermediate/Advanced level, it is important not to approach every exercise with full gusto. If you do, your muscles will become accustomed to that intense level of effort and will quickly accommodate to it and stop strengthening. In addition, these exercises are designed specifically to create lean and toned muscles—not bulked-up muscles. This is basically the same philosophy that you've already learned about overdoing your cardio exercise. Sometimes less really is more!

Interspersing exercises done at the Beginner/Intermediate level with more advanced exercises is a technique I've learned as a bodybuilder, and is the ideal way to confuse your muscles so they work at maximum efficiency every time.

Here are the ways you can mix it up:

I REALLY MISS MY CARDIO! HELP!

As you read in chapter 7, cardio is not the way to lose weight. But it's still good for your cardiovascular system, lungs, and circulation; can make you feel good; and can relieve stress.

If you're used to doing a lot of cardio and are finding the transition difficult, try to stick to this new schedule for at least six weeks. Then do a new body assessment. If you're still craving the cardio—and have seen visible improvements in your shape thanks to the Brown Fat Revolution reshaping—than add a separate day of more cardio. If you add this, you'll be on an eight-day, not a seven-day, schedule.

- Focus on an extremely slow release of the contraction.

- Change the order of the exercises in your circuit.

- Change the number of repetitions; go to fatigue or burn, then push out as many as physically possible beyond that.

- Change the level of the bungee cord's resistance (or the weight of the hand weights).

- Change the reps *and* the weight. For example, you can take a muscle to fatigue by doing fewer reps with more resistance (or weight) on one day; this will stimulate one set of muscle fibers. On another day, you can do multiple reps with a lower resistance (or weight) until there is a burn.

- Use half reps. Half reps take the muscle to fatigue using half the range of motion. For instance, with the biceps, if you did six reps with a full range of motion, your elbow would be opened to 180 degrees. For a half rep, you'd do as many reps as necessary to get to fatigue by doing the same motion but stopping at 90 degrees.

- You can mix up half reps even more by making them start either at the top or the bottom of the range of motion. For example, for the biceps movement described in the above paragraph, if you start with the elbow at 90 degrees and flex it up to the shoulder, this is the top half rep. If you start with the arm at 180 degrees and flex up to 90 degrees, this is the bottom half rep.

- Use the pyramid technique. This involves starting with a higher resistance (or weight) and decreasing it until you reach the burn. So for a biceps curl, you'd pick a bungee cord (or weight) that allows you to get to a burn with eight reps, then without stopping change the cord to another cord with a lower resistance (or drop the weight a few pounds) and do as many reps as possible, then drop it down again to a lower resistance (or weight) and do as many reps as possible. You'll keep going until you cannot do even two reps because the biceps will be completely fatigued.

- Do supersets. In a superset, you'll pick two or three exercises for a muscle, and do one set of each in succession, with no breaks.

- Do circuits. This is when you go from one muscle group to the next without any break.

- Follow training cycles. Unlike trainers or exercise instructors who insist that you work at full throttle at every session, every day, every time—creating way too much stress for your muscles and often leading to injuries or burnout—I strongly believe that exercise should be an expression of what's going on in your brain, too. This means that you should follow the energy of your day. If you've had an especially stressful day at work and feel particularly motivated to get rid of this stress, you can crank it up a notch and use more half reps, pyramids, and supersets. (Or if you're used to working out at the advanced level, but your stressful day at work has drained you of energy to think, you can easily crank it down a notch and go back to an easier level.)

CORE DAY I—ABDOMEN AND SHOULDERS

ABDOMEN

UPPER ABDOMEN

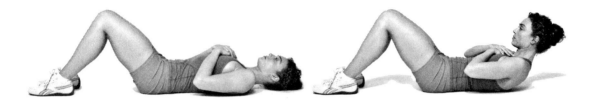

BASIC CRUNCH

1. Lie flat on your back on the floor with your knees bent, arms folded on your chest.

2. Slowly raise your shoulders up toward your pelvis, contracting your abdominal muscles as you do. Keep your chin up and your eyes focused forward.

3. Slowly lower yourself back to the floor.

   - Do not put your hands behind your head, as if you do, you can unwittingly engage your neck and arm muscles, not your abs.

   - Do not take the exercise to a full sit-up position. You only have to go from flat on the floor to a 45-degree angle at the hips, just to the point where you feel a muscle contraction.

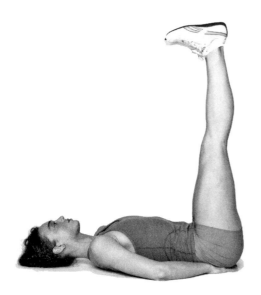 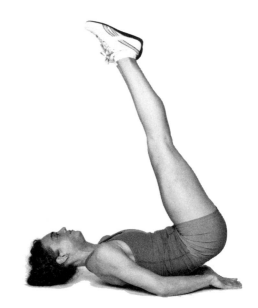

HIP THRUST

1. Lie flat on your back on the floor.

2. Lift your legs straight up, creating a 90-degree angle at the hips.

3. Raise your feet toward the ceiling by pulling your hips up, hold the position, and contract your lower abdominal muscles.

4. Slowly return to starting position.

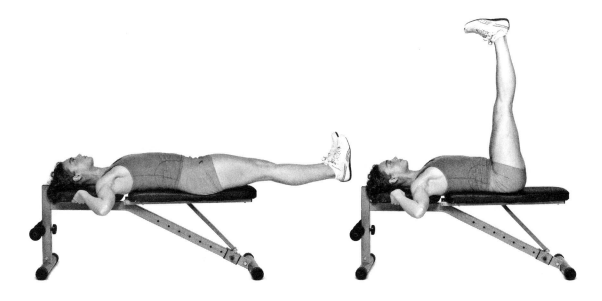

LEG RAISE

1. Lie flat on your back on a bench with your buttocks and knees fully supported. Your legs will extend beyond the edge of the bench.

2. Keep your legs straight and, from your hips, rotate your legs up a full 90 degrees toward the ceiling. You will be creating a 90-degree angle between your feet and your upper body.

3. Slowly lower your legs to starting position.

   - Focus on contracting the abdominal muscles on both the way up and the way down.

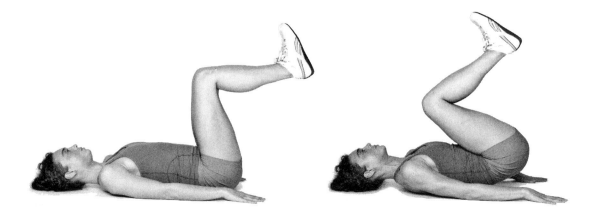

REVERSE CRUNCH

1. Lie on the floor on your back with your legs up, knees bent at 90 degrees.

2. Move your knees toward your chest without changing their position. The arc of rotation comes from your hips and the elevation of your buttocks off the floor. Imagine pulling your belly button up to your pelvis.

3. Hold the abdominals in the flexed position for 10 seconds.

4. Relax the hold and return to starting position.

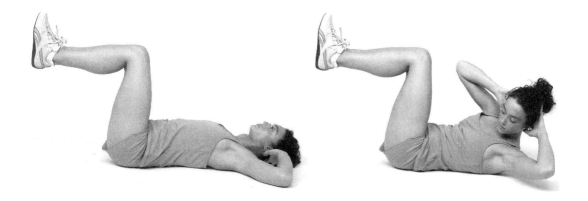

TWISTING CRUNCH

1. Lie on your back and place your hands on the back of your head, behind your ears. Raise your legs and bend them at the knees, at a 90-degree angle.

2. Elevate your shoulders toward your left hip, contract abdominal muscles, and return to resting position.

3. Repeat movement, elevating your shoulders toward your right hip.

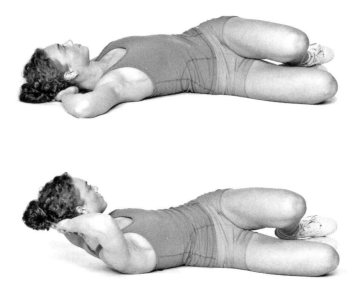

SIDE CRUNCH

1. Lie on your back on the floor, with your legs bent at the knee, then slowly lower your legs to the right, so that your left hip is raised off the floor. Place your hands behind your head.

2. Elevate your shoulders toward your left hip, contract abdominal muscles, and return to resting position.

3. Repeat on opposite side.

FRONT SHOULDERS

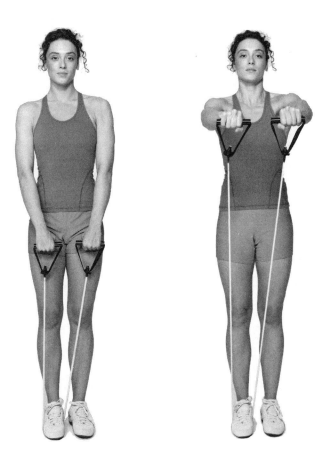

FRONT RAISE—BUNGEE

1. Stand straight, feet together, with a bungee cord securely under one foot and a handle in each hand, arms held loosely down in front of your thighs.

2. Keeping them straight, raise both arms together up to shoulder level.

3. Return to starting position.

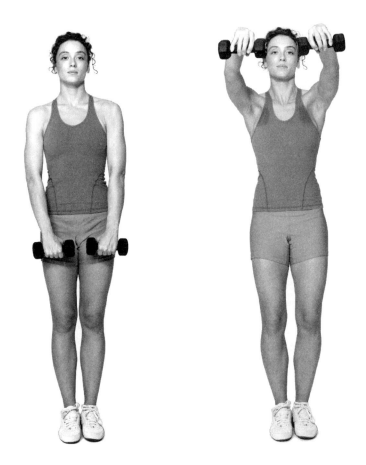

FRONT RAISE—HAND WEIGHTS

1. Hold a hand weight in each hand, palms down, arms held loosely down in front of your thighs.

2. Keeping them straight, raise both arms together up to shoulder level.

3. Return to starting position.

THE BROWN FAT REVOLUTION EXERCISE PLAN

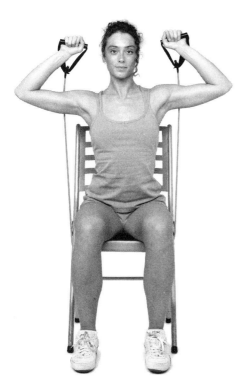
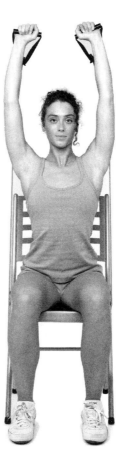

SHOULDER PRESS—BUNGEE

1. Sit erect on a chair or bench, feet shoulder-width apart, with a bungee cord securely under your feet and a handle in each hand. Lift the cord above your shoulders, hands by your head.

2. Lift the bungee in one movement above your head, creating a U.

3. Return to starting position.

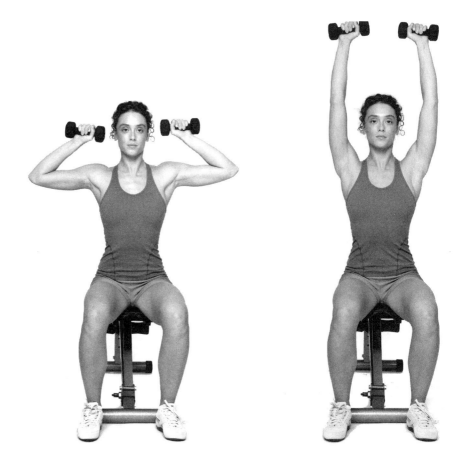

SHOULDER PRESS—HAND WEIGHTS

1. Sit erect on a chair or bench, feet flat on the floor, with a hand weight in each hand, palms facing forward.

2. Lift weights above your shoulders, and then together lift them straight above your head, creating a U with the movement.

3. Return to starting position with weights facing forward.

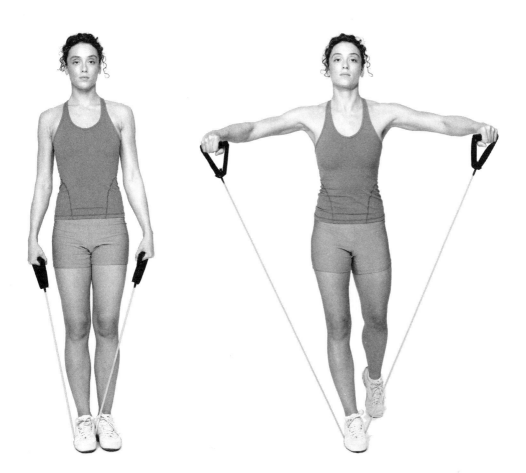

LATERAL RAISE—BUNGEE

1. Stand straight with a bungee cord securely under your right foot and a handle in each hand, palms facing each other at hip level, then lean forward about 10 degrees, feet together, or free foot behind you for stability.

2. Lift your hands out with arms slightly bent at the elbows, as if you were flying, and contract shoulder muscles.

3. Return to starting position.

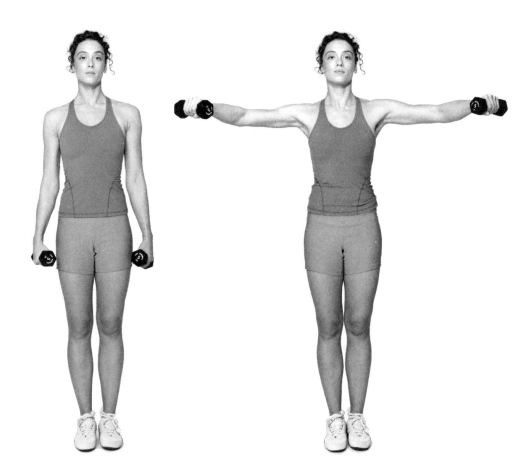

LATERAL RAISE—HAND WEIGHTS

1. Stand straight, then lean forward about 10 degrees, feet together, with a hand weight in each hand, palms facing each other and at hip level.

2. Lift your hands out with arms slightly bent at the elbows, as if you were flying, and contract shoulder muscles.

3. Return to starting position.

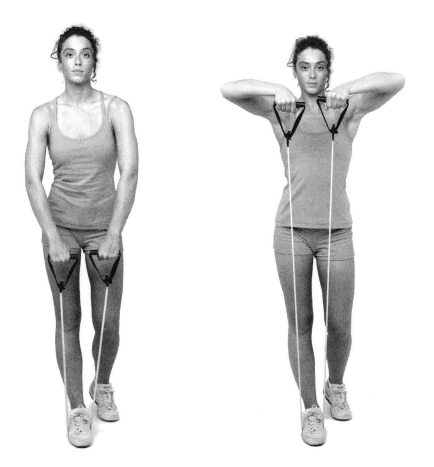

STRAIGHT-UP ROW—BUNGEE

1. Stand straight, right foot forward, with a bungee cord securely under it.

2. Grasp the handles of the cord, palms facing the floor, then pull them up to shoulder level, with arms flexed at the elbow, and contract shoulder muscles.

3. Return to starting position.

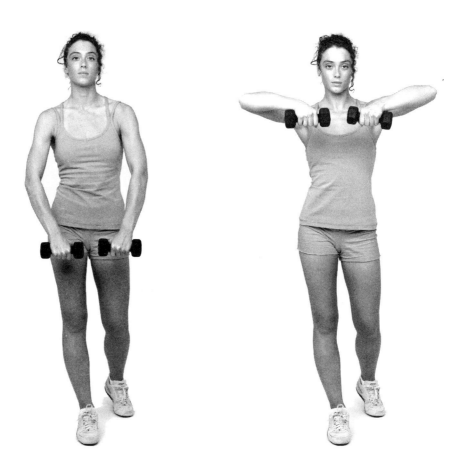

STRAIGHT-UP ROW—HAND WEIGHTS

1. Stand straight, right foot forward, with a hand weight in each hand, palms down. The weights should be at thigh level.

2. Lift weights together to shoulder level, elbows bent, contracting shoulder muscles.

3. Return to starting position.

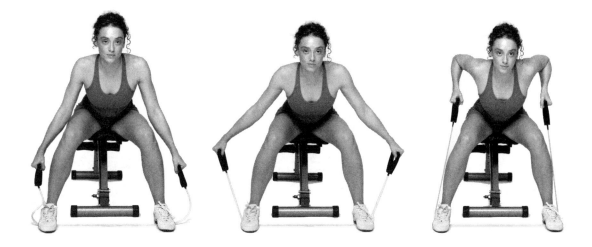

BENT ROW—BUNGEE

1. Sit on a bench or chair, then bend forward so that your chest is almost touching the front of your thighs, with a bungee cord securely under your feet, which should be far apart.

2. Grasp the handles of the cord, palms facing inward.

3. Lift the cord, keeping your elbows close to your sides until your elbows are flexed to 90 degrees, and contract the rear delts (back of shoulders) and upper back.

4. Slowly return to starting position.

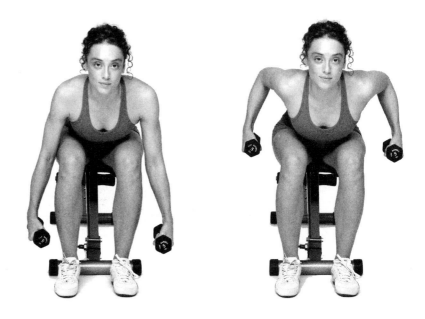

BENT ROW—HAND WEIGHTS

1. Sit on a bench or chair, then bend forward so that your chest is almost touching your thighs.

2. Grasp hand weights, palms facing in.

3. Lift the weights with your elbows flexed to 90 degrees at your sides, and contract rear delts (back of the shoulders) and upper back.

4. Slowly return to starting position.

EXTREMITIES DAY—BICEPS, TRICEPS, AND CALVES

BICEPS

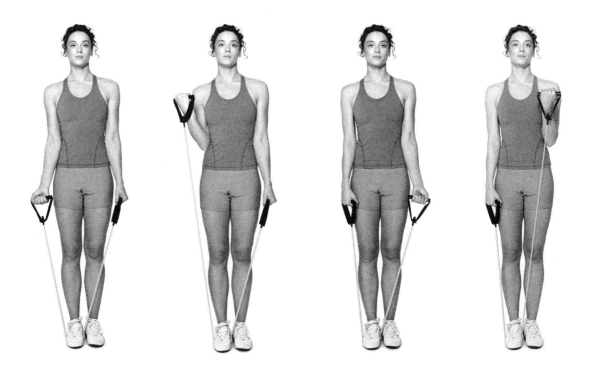

ALTERNATING CURL—BUNGEE

1. Stand straight, feet together, with a bungee cord securely under your right foot.

2. Grasp the handles of the cord with your hands, palms up, elbow held against the body.

3. With your right arm, pull the cord up toward your right shoulder, flexing your arm and contracting your biceps.

4. Hold in full contraction, then release slowly to starting position.

5. Repeat with left arm.

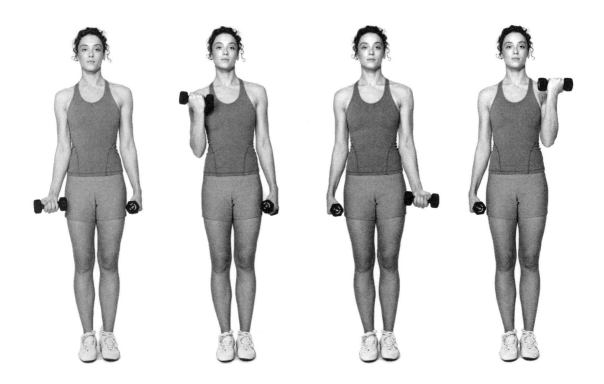

ALTERNATING CURL—HAND WEIGHTS

1. Stand straight, feet together, with a hand weight in each hand, palms facing up, elbows held against the body.

2. Flex your right arm, bringing the weight to shoulder level, contracting your biceps.

3. Hold in full contraction, then release slowly to starting position.

4. Repeat with left arm.

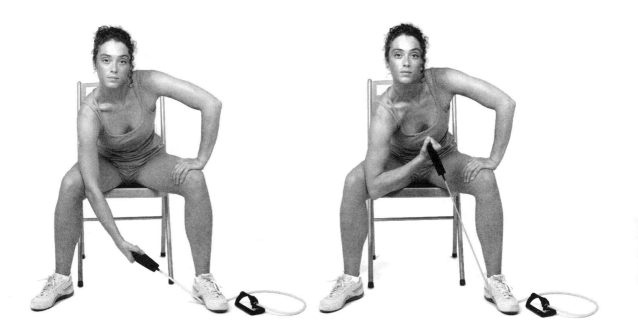

CONCENTRATION CURL—BUNGEE

1. Sit on a chair or bench, feet wide apart, with the bungee cord handle palm up in your right hand, and the midportion of the cord securely fixed under your left foot.

2. Place your right elbow against your right knee.

3. Flex your arm, bringing the handle of the bungee toward your shoulder, contracting your biceps.

4. Hold the contraction, then release slowly to starting position.

5. Perform a full set with your right arm.

6. Repeat with your left arm.

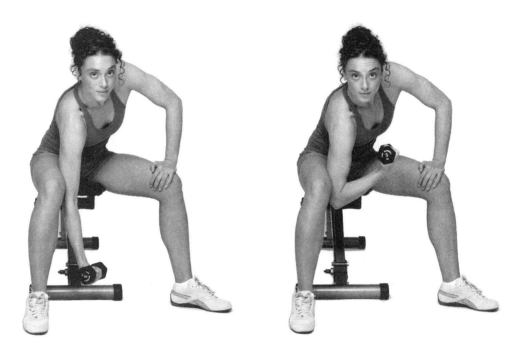

CONCENTRATION CURL—HAND WEIGHTS

1. Sit on a chair or bench, feet wide apart, with a hand weight in your right hand, palm facing up.

2. Place your right elbow against your right knee.

3. Flex your right arm, bringing the weight toward your right shoulder, contracting your biceps.

4. Hold the contraction, then release slowly to starting position.

5. Perform a full set with your right arm.

6. Repeat with your left arm.

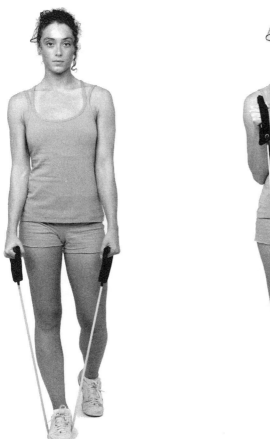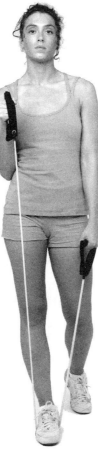

HAMMER CURL—BUNGEE

1. Stand straight, one foot in front of the other, with the bungee cord under your right foot, a handle in each hand, palms facing inward.

2. Flex your right arm, bringing the handle to shoulder level, contracting your biceps.

3. Hold in full contraction, then release slowly to starting position.

4. Repeat with your left arm.

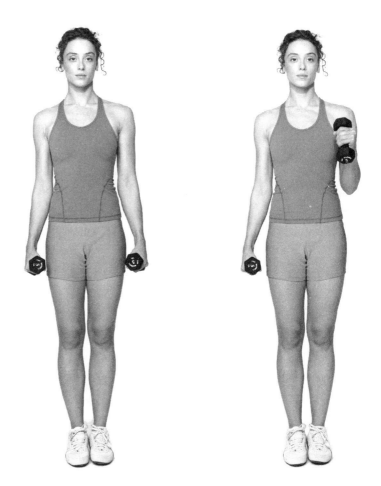

HAMMER CURL—HAND WEIGHTS

1. Stand straight, feet together, with a hand weight in each hand, palms facing inward, elbows held against the body.

2. Flex your left arm, bringing the weight to shoulder level, contracting your biceps.

3. Hold in full contraction, then release slowly to starting position.

4. Repeat with your right arm.

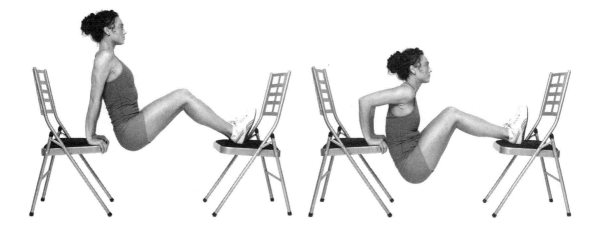

BENCH OR CHAIR DIP

1. Place two benches or chairs half a body length apart, facing each other.

2. Sit at the edge of one with half of your buttocks off the bench/chair, knees flexed at 90 degrees, arms at shoulder width, with hands holding the bench/chair. Your hands should be flat, and facing behind you, gripping the edge of the chair.

3. Secure this position, then place your heels on the opposite bench/chair. Your body should be level with the two benches/chairs.

4. Push off the chair and lower your body as low as you can go by flexing your arms at the elbow.

5. Return to starting position.

   • Make sure to do this exercise with the power of your triceps, not your legs.

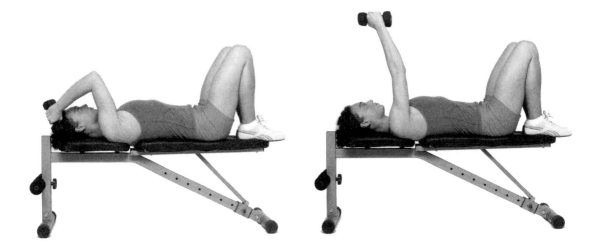

LYING EXTENSION—HAND WEIGHTS

1. Lie flat on a bench with a hand weight in each hand, hands down by your sides and facing each other.

2. Lift weights over your head, then fully flex your elbows so weights move back toward the outside of your ears. Keep your elbows close to your head.

3. Straighten your arms to full extension.

4. Return to starting position.

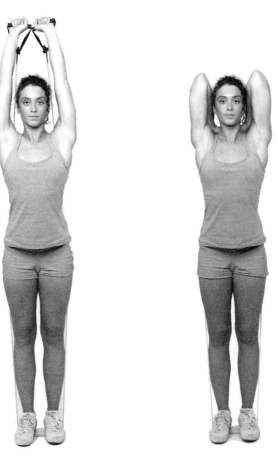

OVERHEAD EXTENSION—BUNGEE

1. Stand straight, feet together, with a bungee cord securely under your feet.

2. Grasp the handles of the cord and lift them above your head.

3. Flex your elbows so that the bungee handles go behind your shoulders (backward). Your elbows should be secured against the sides of your head.

4. Let your hands fall back toward your waist, as far as possible, then pull handles up to the ceiling.

5. Return to starting position.

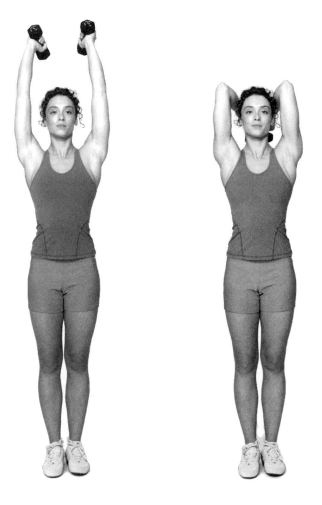

OVERHEAD TWO-ARM EXTENSION—HAND WEIGHTS

1. Stand straight, feet together, with a hand weight in each hand, palms facing each other.

2. Flex your elbows and bring them up to each side of your head, with the weights heading backward.

3. Lower the weights toward your back, then lift them above your head to almost fully extend the arm.

4. Return to starting position.

THE BROWN FAT REVOLUTION EXERCISE PLAN

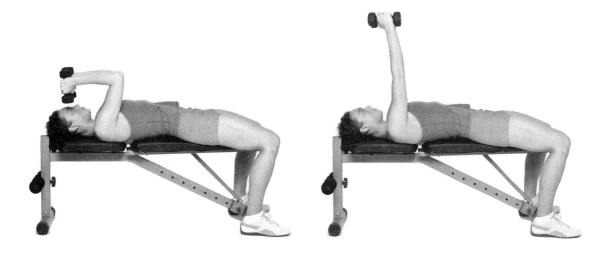

NOSE BREAKER

1. Lie flat on a bench with a hand weight in each hand, palms close and weights almost touching your forehead.

2. Lift weights over your head by straightening your arms up, palms still facing each other, then bend your elbows and bring the weights back, toward your ears.

3. Lower the weights down to a few inches above your nose, then return your arms to starting position.

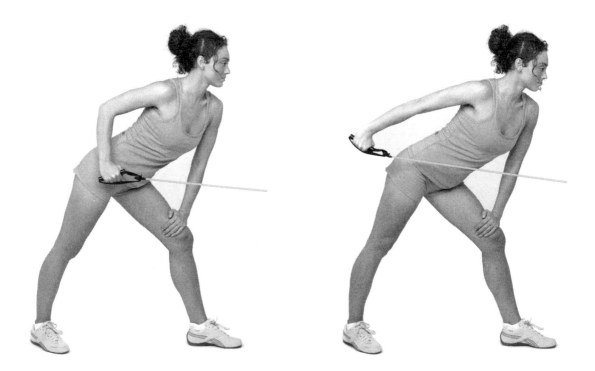

KICKBACK—BUNGEE

1. Secure the bungee cord to a piece of furniture or the door anchor strap by looping the handles through the strap and taking the free handle in your right hand.

2. Bend over 45 degrees at the waist with your left arm resting on your left knee for support. Your right palm should be facing your side, elbow flexed.

3. Fully extend your right arm behind you, raising the bungee handle toward your buttocks, then contract the triceps.

4. Return to starting position.

5. Do one full set with your right arm, then switch to your left arm.

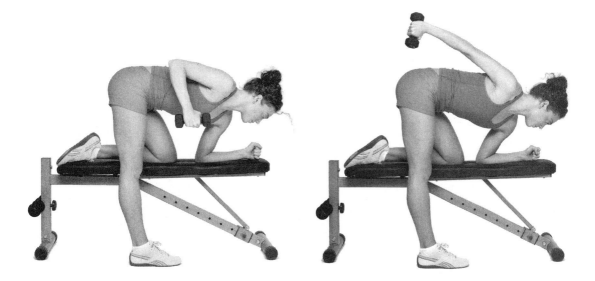

KICKBACK—HAND WEIGHTS

1. With your left knee and left arm resting on a bench or armless chair, bend over so that your back is parallel with the ground. Hold hand weight in your right hand, palm inside, and elbow flexed.

2. Fully extend your arm behind you, raising the weight over your buttocks, using your triceps.

3. Return to starting position with your hand at the side of your chest.

4. Do one full set with your right arm, then switch to your left arm.

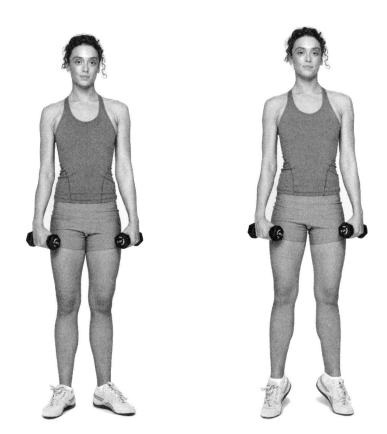

ANGLED CALF RAISE—HAND WEIGHTS

1. Stand straight, feet shoulder-width apart and toes pointing 45 degrees outward, with a hand weight in each hand.

2. Keeping your legs and body straight, stand on your tiptoes, as high as possible, then hold this position for a count of five.

3. Return to starting position.

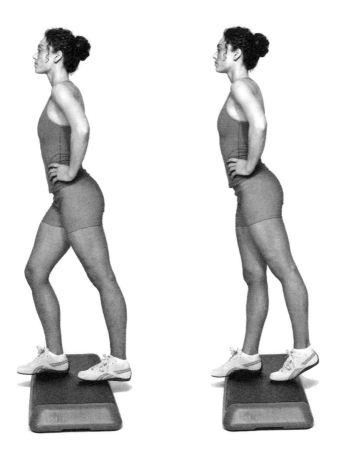

ALTERNATING STAIR RAISE

1. Stand with your left foot on the back edge of a platform or stair. The edge should be halfway under your foot so that your insole is completely supporting you.

2. Lift your left foot on tiptoe, keeping your legs perfectly straight, contracting the calf muscle at the top of the movement. Do not bounce.

3. Do a full set, then switch to the other leg.

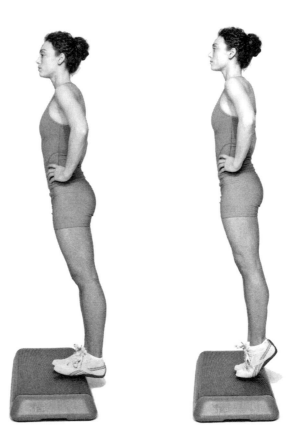

STANDING STAIR RAISE

1. Stand with both feet on the back edge of a platform or stair. The edge of the stair should be halfway under your feet so that your insoles are completely supporting you.

2. Stand on your tiptoes, keeping your legs perfectly straight, contracting the calf muscles at the top of the movement. Do not bounce.

3. Do a full set before returning to starting position.

   • Both Stair Raises can be done holding weights.

GLUTES/HAMSTRINGS

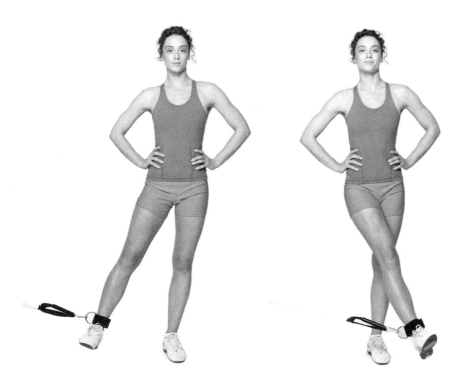

ADDUCTION—BUNGEE

1. Attach one handle of the bungee cord to the door anchor strap or a secure piece of furniture.

2. Attach the other bungee handle to your right ankle strap. The door should be to your right.

3. Raise your right foot forward and then across your left leg. Keep your leg straight at all times.

4. Hold the contraction, then return your right leg to a relaxed position.

5. Do a full set, then switch to your left leg.

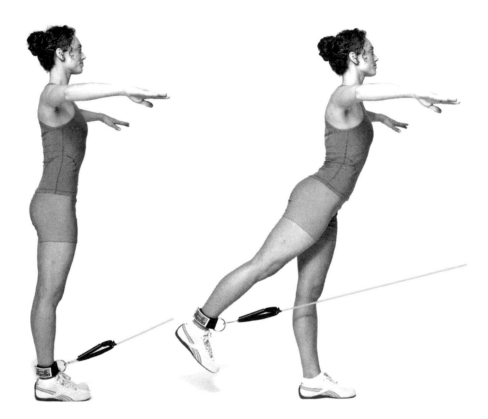

BACK KICK—BUNGEE

1. Attach one handle of the bungee cord to the door anchor strap or a secure piece of furniture.

2. Attach the other bungee handle to your right ankle strap.

3. With arms raised for support, kick back your almost-straight right leg to full extension.

4. Hold the contraction, then slowly release to starting position.

5. Do a full set, then switch to your left leg.

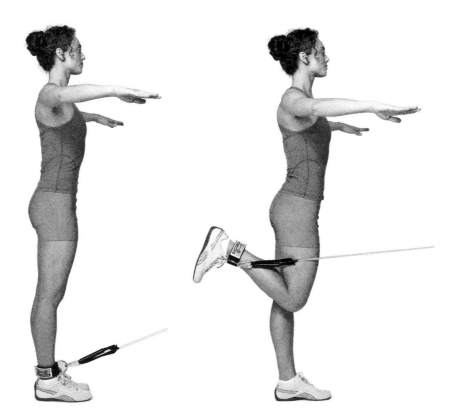

LEG CURL—BUNGEE

1. Attach one handle of the bungee cord to the door anchor strap or a secure piece of furniture.

2. Attach the other bungee handle to your right ankle strap.

3. With arms raised for support, bend your knee back to full flexion (your foot toward your buttocks).

4. Hold the contraction, then slowly release to starting position.

5. Do a full set, then switch to your left leg.

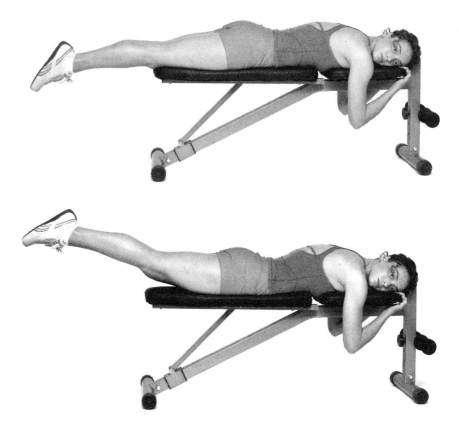

REVERSE HYPEREXTENSION

1. Lie facedown on a firm bed or a flat bench, with the edge around your knees.

2. Lift your legs as high as possible, keeping them straight and the toes pointed.

3. Hold the contraction, then slowly release to starting position.

QUADS AND LOWER BACK

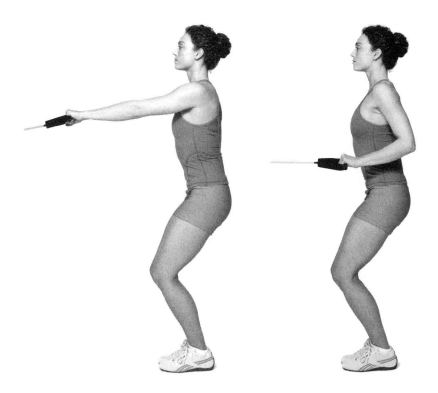

DOUBLE-ARM ROW—BUNGEE

1. Place two bungee cords under a heavy piece of furniture.

2. Stand far enough away that pulling the bungee will cause stretching.

3. Grasp the handles in each hand, palms down, and pull toward your waist, aiming your elbows toward your back.

4. Hold the contraction, then slowly release to starting position.

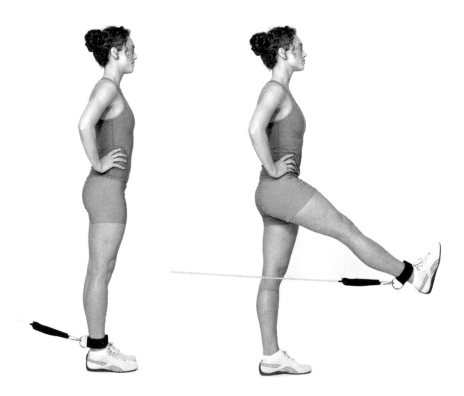

FRONT KICK—BUNGEE

1. Attach one handle of the bungee cord to the door anchor strap or a secure piece of furniture.

2. Attach the other bungee handle to your right ankle strap and stand facing away.

3. With your hands at your waist, move your right leg up slowly to 45 degrees. Keep it straight at all times.

4. Hold the contraction, then slowly release to starting position.

5. Do a full set, then switch to your left leg.

   - Do not move your leg farther than 45 degrees, as this will work your pelvis, not your quads.

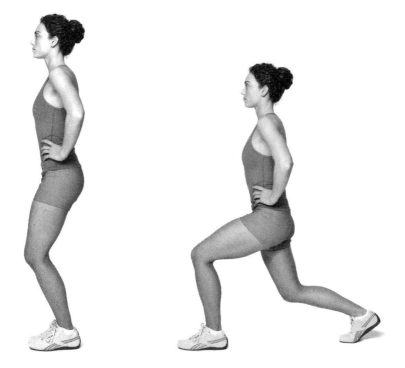

WALKING LUNGE—WITH OR WITHOUT HAND WEIGHTS

1. Stand with your knees bent, arms on waist, feet shoulder-width apart.

2. Step forward about 3 feet with your left foot, bending your right knee down as far as is comfortable. Your left knee should always remain at a 90-degree angle to the floor, and never move in front of your foot. Keep your toes pointed out about 45 degrees for stability.

3. Return to starting position.

4. Repeat with your right leg.

   • This exercise can be done with or without hand weights. Remember to always start without weights until you're confident with the movement. The Walking Lunge not only works your glutes and quads, but enlists several core muscles for balance and stability.

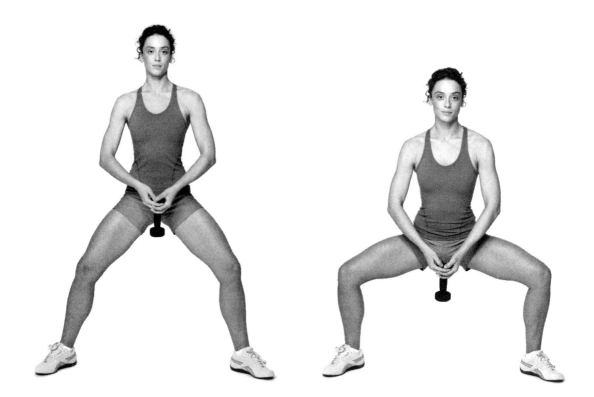

PLIÉ SQUAT—HAND WEIGHTS

1. Stand straight, with your feet wide apart, toes pointing 45 degrees outward, with a hand weight held in front of your body, elbows slightly bent.

2. As if you were about to sit down into a chair, lower your buttocks toward the floor until your thighs are parallel with the floor.

3. Return to starting position and repeat.

   • Make sure your feet are more than hip-width apart.

   • Make sure you keep your back straight as you go down. Do not arch forward.

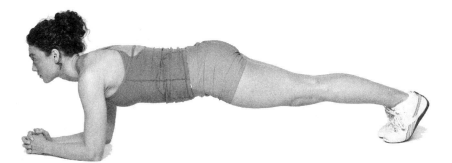

ABDOMEN STRETCH (PLANK)

1. Lie on your belly on the floor, palms together, forearms and elbows flat on the floor, elbows bent to 90 degrees.

2. Lift your body onto your elbows and keep it horizontal from the shoulders to the heels.

3. Hold this position, keeping as still as possible for as long as you can while still maintaining perfect form.

4. Return to starting position. Repeat 3 times.

   - Focus on contracting your core while maintaining relaxed breathing.

   - At first, you will not be able to hold the position for very long—perhaps not even 10 seconds—but your strength and stamina will increase the more you do this exercise.

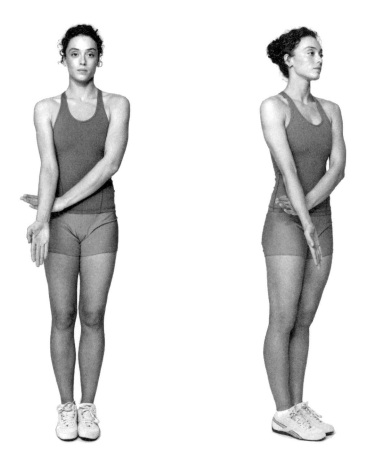

BICEPS STRETCH

1. Stand straight with your right arm stretched out away from you, palm facing out.

2. Put your left hand behind and below your right elbow, then use the leverage of your left hand to push your right forearm forward.

3. Resist this forward movement by focusing on moving your right hand back toward your body.

4. Hold the position for 20 seconds, feeling the stretch in the biceps.

5. Repeat with your left arm supported by your right arm.

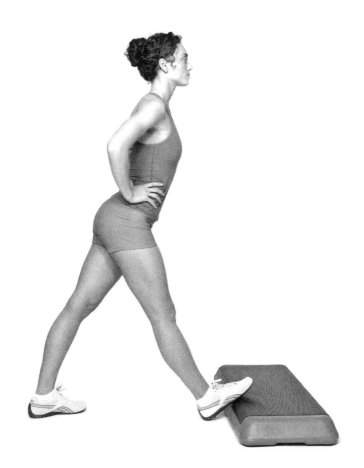

CALF STRETCH

1. Place the insole of your right foot on the edge of a platform or stair, with your heel hanging off.

2. Bend your left leg and shift all your weight onto your right foot, letting your right heel fall toward the floor. You will feel the stretch in your calf.

3. Hold for 20 seconds.

4. Repeat with the other leg.

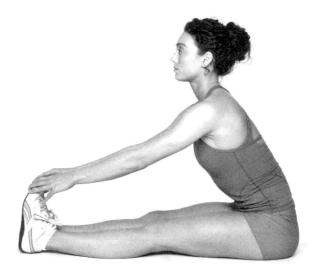

HAMSTRING STRETCH

1. Sit on the floor with your legs fully extended, toes pointed to the ceiling.

2. Grab your knees and then move your hands slowly toward your toes. Take them as far as they can go, feeling the pull in your hamstrings.

3. Hold for at least 20 seconds, or as long as you can.

4. Relax and return to starting position. Repeat 3 times.

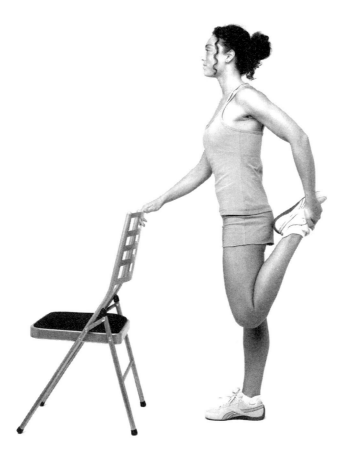

QUADS STRETCH

1. Stand straight, facing a table or chair back to hold on to with your right hand.

2. Bend your left knee, then grab your left foot with your left hand and push that foot toward your buttocks. Feel the stretch.

3. Hold for 20 seconds, or as long as you can.

4. Release and repeat with the other side, holding on with your left hand and working your right leg.

5. Do 3 reps, alternating sides, for each quads.

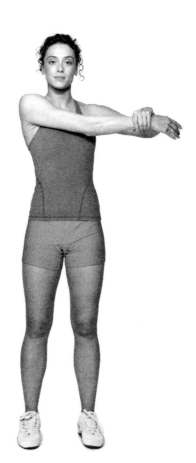

SHOULDER STRETCH

1. Stand straight in front of a mirror, feet shoulder-width apart.

2. Keep your body facing forward, then pull your right arm across your chest with your left hand.

3. Hold the position for 10 seconds, then slowly release.

4. Repeat with the left arm.

5. Do 3 reps, alternating sides, for each shoulder.

THE BROWN FAT REVOLUTION EXERCISE PLAN

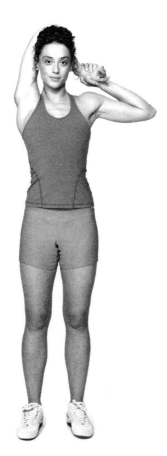

TRICEPS STRETCH

1. With your hands over your head, grab your right wrist with your left hand and pull your right arm over your head to the left.

2. Hold for 20 seconds.

3. Repeat with the other side.

9.
FOUR-WEEK EXERCISE PLAN FOR THE HORMONE CATEGORY I— BEGINNER/INTERMEDIATE

WEEKLY CYCLE

DAY 1: CORE DAY I

Abdomen
Shoulders

DAY 2: EXTREMITIES DAY

Biceps
Triceps
Calves

DAY 3: CORE DAY II

Glutes
Hamstrings

DAY 4: CORE DAY III

Quads
Lower Back

DAY 5: CARDIO DAY

No more than 30 minutes of "sprinted" cardio

DAY 6: OFF DAY

DAY 7: OFF DAY

FOUR-WEEK SCHEDULE

Once you've mastered these routines, you can mix them up with different selections from the exercises listed in chapter 8.

DAY 1: CORE DAY I

Start with 2–3 minutes of stretching your shoulders.

Sit on an armless chair, with back erect, shoulders back, heels flat against the floor, knees bent at 90 degrees, and hands on knees. You should be able to see your toes by simply looking down, without bending. You should also feel long, as if being pulled from the top of your head off your seat, as well as relaxed. Now gently pull your lower abdomen inward toward your back. Do not suck it in—*draw* your belly button into your back. Breathe normally. Hold this posture for 10 seconds. Repeat this 5 times.

You have now engaged your core and are ready to proceed with your Core Curriculum for today.

- Abdomen exercises: Basic Crunch, Leg Raise, Twisting Crunch. Do 10 of each, take a 1-minute break, then do 10 of each.

- Shoulder exercises: Bent Row—Bungee, Lateral Raise—Bungee or Hand Weights, Shoulder Press—Bungee or Hand Weights. Do 3 sets of 10 for each, 1 minute apart.

DAY 2: EXTREMITIES DAY

Start with 5 minutes of stretching your biceps, triceps, and calves. Stretch each for 10 seconds with no break in between muscle groups. Repeat entire set 3 times.

Engage your core, as in Day 1.

- Biceps exercise: Alternating Curl—Bungee. Do 3 sets of 10, 1 minute apart.

- Triceps exercise: Overhead Extension—Bungee, or Lying Extension—Hand Weights. Do 3 sets of 10, 1 minute apart.

- Calves exercise: Standing Stair Raise. Do 3 sets of 10, 1 minute apart. Keep toes pointed inward.

DAY 3: CORE DAY II

Start with 2–3 minutes of stretching your hamstrings.

Engage your core, as in Day 1.

- Glutes exercise: Leg Curl—Bungee. Do 3 sets of 10, 1 minute apart.

- Hamstring exercise: Back Kick—Bungee. Do 3 sets of 10, 1 minute apart.

DAY 4: CORE DAY III

Start with 2–3 minutes of stretching your quads.

Engage your core, as in Day 1.

- Quads exercise: Front Kick—Bungee. Do 3 sets of 10, 1 minute apart.

- Lower back exercise: Double-Arm Row—Bungee. Do 3 sets of 10, 1 minute apart.

DAY 5: CARDIO DAY

Exercise for no more than 30 minutes of "sprinted" cardio.

DAY 6: OFF DAY

DAY 7: OFF DAY

DAY 8: CORE DAY I

Start with 2–3 minutes of stretching your shoulders.

Engage your core, as in Day 1.

- Abdomen exercises: Basic Crunch, Hip Thrust, Side Crunch. Do 3 sets of at least 10 or more (as many as you can do), 1 minute apart.

- Shoulder exercises: Bent Row—Bungee, Lateral Raise—Bungee, Straight-up Row—Bungee. Do 3 sets of 10, 1 minute apart.

DAY 9: EXTREMITIES DAY

Start with 5 minutes of stretching your biceps, triceps, and calves. Stretch each for 10 seconds with no break in between muscle groups. Repeat entire set 3 times.

Engage your core, as in Day 1.

- Biceps exercise: Alternating Curl—Bungee. Do 3 sets of 10, 1 minute apart.

- Triceps exercise: Overhead Two-Arm Extension—Hand Weights, or Bench or Chair Dip. Do 3 sets of 10, 1 minute apart.

- Calves exercise: Angled Calf Raise—Hand Weights. Do 3 sets of 10. Keep feet together.

DAY 10: CORE DAY II

Start with 2–3 minutes of stretching your hamstrings.

Engage your core, as in Day 1.

- Glutes exercise: Back Kick—Bungee. Do 3 sets of 10, 1 minute apart.

- Hamstring exercise: Leg Curl—Bungee. Do 3 sets of 10, 1 minute apart.

DAY 11: CORE DAY III

Start with 2–3 minutes of stretching your quads.

Engage your core, as in Day 1.

- Quads exercise: Front Kick—Bungee. Do 3 sets of 10, 1 minute apart.

- Lower back exercise: Double-Arm Row—Bungee. Do 3 sets of 10, 1 minute apart.

DAY 12: CARDIO DAY

Exercise for no more than 30 minutes of "sprinted" cardio.

DAY 13: OFF DAY

DAY 14: OFF DAY

DAY 15: CORE DAY I

Start with 2–3 minutes of stretching your shoulders.

Engage your core, as in Day 1.

- Abdomen exercises: Basic Crunch, Reverse Crunch, Side Crunch. Do 10 of each, take a 1-minute break, then do 10 of each.

- Shoulder exercises: Bent Row—Bungee, Lateral Raise— Bungee, Straight-up Row—Bungee. Do 3 sets of 10, 1 minute apart.

DAY 16: EXTREMITIES DAY

Start with 5 minutes of stretching your biceps, triceps, and calves. Stretch each for 10 seconds with no break in between muscle groups. Repeat entire set 3 times.

Engage your core, as in Day 1.

- Biceps exercise: Alternating Curl—Bungee. Do 3 sets of 10, 1 minute apart.

- Triceps exercise: Kickback—Bungee or Hand Weights, or Overhead Extension—Bungee. Do 3 sets of 10, 1 minute apart.

- Calves exercise: Alternating Stair Raise. Do 3 sets of 10, 1 minute apart.

DAY 17: CORE DAY II

Start with 2–3 minutes of stretching your hamstrings.

Engage your core, as in Day 1.

- Glutes exercise: Adduction—Bungee. Do 3 sets of 10, 1 minute apart.

- Hamstring exercise: Reverse Hyperextension. Do 3 sets of 10, 1 minute apart.

DAY 18: CORE DAY III

Start with 2–3 minutes of stretching your quads.

Engage your core, as in Day 1.

- Quads exercise: Walking Lunge. Do 5 steps forward, 5 steps back, rest 1 minute, and repeat for a total of three sets.

- Lower back exercise: Double-Arm Row—Bungee. Do 3 sets of 10, 1 minute apart.

DAY 19: CARDIO DAY

Exercise for no more than 30 minutes of "sprinted" cardio.

DAY 20: OFF DAY

DAY 21: OFF DAY

DAY 22: CORE DAY I

Start with 2–3 minutes of stretching your shoulders.

Engage your core, as in Day 1.

- Abdomen exercises: Basic Crunch, Leg Raise, Side Crunch. Do 3 sets of at least 10 or more (as many as you can do), 1 minute apart.

- Shoulder exercises: Bent Row—Bungee, Front Raise— Bungee or Hand Weights, Lateral Raise—Bungee or Hand Weights. Do 3 sets of 10, 1 minute apart.

DAY 23: EXTREMITIES DAY

Start with 5 minutes of stretching your biceps, triceps, and calves. Stretch each for 10 seconds with no break in between muscle groups. Repeat entire set 3 times.

Engage your core, as in Day 1.

- Biceps exercise: Alternating Curl—Bungee. Do 3 sets of 10, 1 minute apart.

- Triceps exercise: Kickback—Bungee or Hand Weights, or Bench or Chair Dip. Do 3 sets of 10, 1 minute apart.

- Calves exercise: Angled Calf Raise—With or Without Hand Weights. Do 3 sets of 10, 1 minute apart.

DAY 24: CORE DAY II

Start with 2–3 minutes of stretching your glutes.

Engage your core, as in Day 1.

- Glutes exercise: Adduction—Bungee. Do 3 sets of 10, 1 minute apart.

- Hamstring exercise: Leg Curl—Bungee. Do 3 sets of 10, 1 minute apart.

DAY 25: CORE DAY III

Start with 2–3 minutes of stretching your quads.

Engage your core, as in Day 1.

- Quads exercise: Plié Squat—With or Without Hand Weights. Do 3 sets of 10, 1 minute apart.

- Lower back exercise: Double-Arm Row—Bungee. Do 3 sets of 10, 1 minute apart.

DAY 26: CARDIO DAY

Exercise for no more than 30 minutes of "sprinted" cardio.

DAY 27: OFF DAY

DAY 28: OFF DAY

MONITORING YOUR PROGRESS

Body shaping occurs gradually, so it can be very helpful to monitor your progress by measuring yourself at the beginning of your program and at the end of each week. If you do want to keep tabs as you transform yourself, this table should help.

MEASUREMENT	START	WEEK 1	WEEK 2	WEEK 3	WEEK 4
WEIGHT					
WAIST					
HIPS					
UPPER ARMS					

10.
FOUR-WEEK EXERCISE PLAN FOR THE HORMONE CATEGORY I— INTERMEDIATE/ADVANCED

WEEKLY CYCLE

DAY 1: CORE DAY I

Abdomen
Shoulders

DAY 2: EXTREMITIES DAY

Biceps
Triceps
Calves

DAY 3: CORE DAY II

Glutes
Hamstrings

DAY 4: CORE DAY III

Quads
Lower Back

DAY 5: CARDIO DAY

No more than 30 minutes of "sprinted" cardio

DAY 6: OFF DAY

DAY 7: OFF DAY

FOUR-WEEK SCHEDULE

Once you've mastered these routines, you can mix them up with different selections from the exercises listed in chapter 8.

DAY 1: CORE DAY I

Start with 2–3 minutes of stretching your shoulders.

Sit on an armless chair, with back erect, shoulders back, heels flat against the floor, knees bent at 90 degrees, and hands on knees. You should be able to see your toes by simply looking down, without bending. You should also feel long, as if being pulled from the top of your head off your seat, as well as relaxed. Now gently pull your lower abdomen inward toward your back. Do not suck it in—*draw* your belly button into your back. Breathe normally. Hold this posture for 10 seconds. Repeat this 5 times.

You have now engaged your core and are ready to proceed with your Core Curriculum for today.

- Abdomen exercises: Basic Crunch, Leg Raise, Side Crunch. Superset: Do 10 of each exercise without resting. Rest 2 minutes. Do 3 supersets.

- Shoulder exercises: Bent Row—Bungee, Shoulder Press—Bungee, Front Raise—Bungee. Do 1 set of 10 each without any rest. Rest 2 minutes and repeat for 3 supersets total, 1 minute apart.

DAY 2: EXTREMITIES DAY

Start with 5 minutes of stretching your biceps, triceps, and calves. Stretch each for 10 seconds with no break in between muscle groups. Repeat entire set 3 times.

Engage your core, as in Day 1.

- Biceps exercise: Concentration Curl—Bungee. Pyramid: Do 10 reps with a heavy bungee cord. Immediately drop down to next resistance-cord level, do 10 reps, immediately drop it again to next level, and do as many reps as you can to bring muscle to full fatigue.

- Triceps exercise: Overhead Extension—Bungee, or Lying Extension—Hand Weights. Do 3 sets of 10 with a full range of motion, followed by 10 half reps (top) per set, 1 minute apart.

- Calves exercise: Standing Stair Raise. Do 3 sets of as many as possible, 1 minute apart. Keep toes pointed inward.

DAY 3: CORE DAY II

Start with 2–3 minutes of stretching your hamstrings.

Engage your core, as in Day 1.

- Glutes exercise: Back Kick—Bungee.

- Hamstring exercise: Leg Curl—Bungee. Circuit: Do 1 set of 10 Back Kicks and 1 set of 10 Leg Curls without any rest. Rest 2 minutes. Do 3 circuits.

DAY 4: CORE DAY III

Start with 2–3 minutes of stretching your quads.

Engage your core, as in Day 1.

- Quads exercise: Front Kick—Bungee. Do with heaviest possible cord resistance.

- Lower back exercises: Double-Arm Row—Bungee. Do with heaviest possible cord resistance. Circuit: Do 1 set of 10 Front Kicks, immediately followed by 1 set of 10 Double-Arm Rows. Rest 1 minute. Do 2 circuits.

DAY 5: CARDIO DAY

Exercise for no more than 30 minutes of "sprinted" cardio.

DAY 6: OFF DAY

DAY 7: OFF DAY

DAY 8: CORE DAY I

Start with 2–3 minutes of stretching your shoulders.

Engage your core, as in Day 1.

- Abdomen exercises: Basic Crunch, Hip Thrust, Side Crunch. Superset: Do 10 of each exercise without resting. Rest 2 minutes. Do 3 supersets.

- Shoulder exercises: Bent Row—Bungee, Lateral Raise— Bungee, Straight-up Row—Bungee. Do 3 sets of 10, 1 minute apart.

DAY 9: EXTREMITIES DAY

Start with 5 minutes of stretching your biceps, triceps, and calves. Stretch each for 10 seconds with no break in between muscle groups. Repeat entire set 3 times.

Engage your core, as in Day 1.

- Biceps exercise: Alternating Curl—Bungee. Do 10 reps with a full range of motion, immediately followed by 10 half reps (bottom). Rest 1 minute, then repeat for 3 sets.

- Triceps exercise: Bench or Chair Dip, or Overhead Two-Arm Extension—Hand Weights. Do 3 sets of 10, 1 minute apart.

- Calves exercise: Standing Stair Raise and Alternating Stair Raise. Superset: Do 10 of each exercise without resting. Rest 2 minutes. Do 3 supersets.

DAY 10: CORE DAY II

Start with 2–3 minutes of stretching your hamstrings.

Engage your core, as in Day 1.

THE BROWN FAT REVOLUTION EXERCISE PLAN

- Glutes exercise: Back Kick—Bungee. Do as many reps as possible to take the glutes to burn. Rest 1 minute and repeat for 3 sets.

- Hamstring exercise: Leg Curl—Bungee. Do 3 sets of 10, 1 minute apart.

DAY 11: CORE DAY III

Start with 2–3 minutes of stretching your quads.

Engage your core, as in Day 1.

- Quads exercises: Plié Squat—With or Without Handweights, Walking Lunge—With or Without Hand Weights. Superset: Do 10 Plié Squats followed immediately by 10 Walking Lunges—5 forward and 5 backward. Rest for 2 minutes and repeat.

- Lower back exercise: Double-Arm Row—Bungee. Do 3 sets of 10, 1 minute apart.

DAY 12: CARDIO DAY

Exercise for no more than 30 minutes of "sprinted" cardio.

DAY 13: OFF DAY

DAY 14: OFF DAY

DAY 15: CORE DAY I

Start with 2–3 minutes of stretching your shoulders.

Engage your core, as in Day 1.

- Abdomen exercises: Basic Crunch, Reverse Crunch, Side Crunch. Superset: Do as many as possible of each. Rest 1 minute between sets.

- Shoulder exercises: Front Raise—Bungee, Lateral Raise—Bungee, Straight-up Row—Bungee. Do 3 sets of 10, 1 minute apart.

DAY 16: EXTREMITIES DAY

Start with 5 minutes of stretching your biceps, triceps, and calves. Stretch each for 10 seconds with no break in between muscle groups. Repeat entire set 3 times.

Engage your core, as in Day 1.

- Biceps exercise: Alternating Curl—Bungee. Do 3 sets of 10, 1 minute apart.

- Triceps exercises: Bench or Chair Dip; Kickback—Bungee or Hand Weights, or Overhead Extension—Bungee. Superset: Do 10 of each exercise without resting. Rest 2 minutes. Do 3 supersets.

- Calves exercise: Alternating Stair Raise. Do 3 sets of 10, 1 minute apart. Add hand weights, as heavy as comfortable, in each hand.

DAY 17: CORE DAY II

Start with 2–3 minutes of stretching your hamstrings.

Engage your core, as in Day 1.

- Glutes exercise: Adduction—Bungee. Do 3 sets of 10, 1 minute apart.

- Hamstring exercises: Reverse Hyperextension. Do 3 sets of 10, 1 minute apart. Leg Curl—Bungee. Superset: Do 10 Reverse Hyperextensions followed immediately by 10 Leg Curls—Bungee with each leg. Rest 2 minutes and repeat for 3 supersets.

DAY 18: CORE DAY III

Start with 2–3 minutes of stretching your quads.

Engage your core, as in Day 1.

- Quads exercise: Walking Lunge—With or Without Hand Weights. Do 5 steps forward, 5 steps back, rest 1 minute. Do 3 sets.

- Lower back exercise: Double-Arm Row—Bungee. Do 3 sets of 10, 1 minute apart.

DAY 19: CARDIO DAY

Exercise for no more than 30 minutes of "sprinted" cardio.

DAY 20: OFF DAY

DAY 21: OFF DAY

DAY 22: CORE DAY I

Start with 2–3 minutes of stretching your shoulders.

Engage your core, as in Day 1.

- Abdomen exercises: Basic Crunch, Leg Raise, Side Crunch. Do as many of each exercise as you can possibly do. Rest 1 minute. Do 2 sets.

- Shoulder exercises: Bent Row—Bungee, Front Raise—Bungee, Lateral Raise—Bungee. Superset: Do 10 of each without resting. Rest 2 minutes. Do 3 supersets.

DAY 23: EXTREMITIES DAY

Start with 5 minutes of stretching your biceps, triceps, and calves. Stretch each for 10 seconds with no break in between muscle groups. Repeat entire set 3 times.

Engage your core, as in Day 1.

- Biceps exercise: Alternating Curl—Bungee. Do 10 half reps (top) immediately followed by 10 with a full range of motion. Rest 1 minute. Do 3 sets.

- Triceps exercise: Kickback—Bungee or Hand Weights. Pyramid: Choose heaviest comfortable weight or strongest cord resistance, do 1 set of 10, drop weight or cord resistance to next level, do 10 reps, drop to next level again, and do as many reps as needed to take the triceps to fatigue. Rest 2 minutes and repeat for 3 pyramids.

- Calves exercises: Standing Stair Raise, Alternating Stair Raise. Superset—Do 10 of each exercise without resting. Rest 2 minutes and repeat. Do 3 supersets.

DAY 24: CORE DAY II

Start with 2–3 minutes of stretching your glutes.

Engage your core, as in Day 1.

- Glutes exercise: Adduction—Bungee. Add ankle weights.

- Hamstring exercise: Leg Curl—Bungee. Superset: Do 10 of each exercise without resting. Rest 2 minutes. Do 3 supersets.

DAY 25: CORE DAY III

Start with 2–3 minutes of stretching your quads.

Engage your core, as in Day 1.

- Quads exercises: Front Kick, Walking Lunges—With or Without Hand Weights. Superset: Do 10 Front Kicks, followed immediately by Walking Lunges, 5 steps forward and 5 steps back. Rest 2 minutes and repeat for 3 supersets.

- Lower back exercise: Double-Arm Row—Bungee. Do 3 sets of 10, 1 minute apart.

DAY 26: CARDIO DAY

Exercise for no more than 30 minutes of "sprinted" cardio.

DAY 27: OFF DAY

DAY 28: OFF DAY

MONITORING YOUR PROGRESS

Body shaping occurs gradually, so it can be very helpful to monitor your progress by measuring yourself at the beginning of your program and at the end of each week. If you do want to keep tabs as you transform yourself, this table should help.

MEASUREMENT	START	WEEK 1	WEEK 2	WEEK 3	WEEK 4
WEIGHT					
WAIST					
HIPS					
UPPER ARMS					

11.
FOUR-WEEK EXERCISE PLAN FOR THE HORMONE CATEGORY II— BEGINNER/INTERMEDIATE

Even though you're in the Hormone Category II years, you don't have to resign yourself to "middle-age spread." Because declining hormone levels trigger more fat deposits in the abdomen and in the upper arms, you'll notice that an extra day targeting these areas, particularly the lower abdomen, has been added to the cycle.

WEEKLY CYCLE

DAY 1: CORE DAY I

Abdomen
Shoulders

DAY 2: EXTREMITIES DAY

Biceps
Triceps
Calves

DAY 3: CORE DAY II

Glutes
Hamstrings

DAY 4: CORE DAY III

Quads

Lower Back

DAY 5: CARDIO DAY

No more than 30 minutes of "sprinted" cardio

DAY 6: ABDOMEN/TRICEPS DAY

Abdomen

Triceps

DAY 7: OFF DAY

DAY 8: OFF DAY

FOUR-WEEK SCHEDULE

Once you've mastered these routines, you can mix them up with different selections from the exercises listed in chapter 8.

DAY 1: CORE DAY I

Start with 2–3 minutes of stretching your shoulders.

Sit on an armless chair, with back erect, shoulders back, heels flat against the floor, knees bent at 90 degrees, and hands on knees. You should be able to see your toes by simply looking down, without bending. You should also feel long, as if being pulled from the top of your head off your seat, as well as relaxed. Now gently pull your lower abdomen inward toward your back. Do not suck it in—*draw* your belly button into your back. Breathe normally. Hold this posture for 10 seconds. Repeat this 5 times.

You have now engaged your core and are ready to proceed with your Core Curriculum for today.

- Abdomen exercises: Basic Crunch, Reverse Crunch, Twisting Crunch. Do 10 of each, take a 1-minute break, then do 10 of each.

- Shoulder exercises: Bent Row—Bungee, Lateral Raise—Bungee, Shoulder Press—Bungee. Do 3 sets of 10 for each, 1 minute apart.

DAY 2: EXTREMITIES DAY

Start with 5 minutes of stretching your biceps, triceps, and calves. Stretch each for 10 seconds with no break in between muscle groups. Repeat entire set 3 times.

Engage your core, as in Day 1.

- Biceps exercise: Alternating Curl—Bungee or Hand Weights. Do 3 sets of 10, 1 minute apart.

- Triceps exercise: Overhead Extension—Bungee. Do 3 sets of 10, 1 minute apart.

- Calves exercise: Standing Stair Raise. Do 3 sets of 10, 1 minute apart. Keep toes pointed inward (pigeon-toed).

DAY 3: CORE DAY II

Start with 2–3 minutes of stretching your hamstrings.

Engage your core, as in Day 1.

- Glutes exercise: Leg Curl—Bungee. Do 3 sets of 10, 1 minute apart.

- Hamstring exercise: Back Kick—Bungee. Do 3 sets of 10, 1 minute apart.

DAY 4: CORE DAY III

Start with 2–3 minutes of stretching your quads.

Engage your core, as in Day 1.

- Quads exercise: Front Kick—Bungee. Do 3 sets of 10, 1 minute apart.

- Lower back exercise: Double-Arm Row—Bungee. Do 3 sets of 10, 1 minute apart.

DAY 5: CARDIO DAY

Exercise for no more than 30 minutes of "sprinted" cardio.

DAY 6: ABDOMEN/TRICEPS DAY

Start with 2–3 minutes of stretching your abdomen and triceps.

Engage your core, as in Day 1.

- Abdomen exercises: Basic Crunch, Hip Thrust, Leg Raise. Do 10 of each, take a 1-minute break, then do 10 more of each.

- Triceps exercise: Bench or Chair Dip. Do 3 sets of 10, 1 minute apart.

DAY 7: OFF DAY

DAY 8: OFF DAY

DAY 9: CORE DAY I

Start with 2–3 minutes of stretching your shoulders.

Engage your core, as in Day 1.

- Abdomen exercises: Basic Crunch, Hip Thrust, Side Crunch. Do 3 sets of at least 10 or more (as many as you can do), 1 minute apart.

- Shoulder exercises: Bent Row—Bungee, Lateral Raise—Bungee, Straight-up Row—Bungee. Do 3 sets of 10, 1 minute apart.

DAY 10: EXTREMITIES DAY

Start with 5 minutes of stretching your biceps, triceps, and calves. Stretch each for 10 seconds with no break in between muscle groups. Repeat entire set 3 times.

Engage your core, as in Day 1.

- Biceps exercise: Alternating Curl—Bungee. Do 3 sets of 10, 1 minute apart.

- Triceps exercise: Overhead Extension—Bungee. Do 3 sets of 10, 1 minute apart.

- Calves exercise: Angled Calf Raise—Hand Weights. Do 3 sets of 10. Keep feet together.

DAY 11: CORE DAY II

Start with 2–3 minutes of stretching your hamstrings.

Engage your core, as in Day 1.

- Glutes exercise: Back Kick—Bungee. Do 3 sets of 10, 1 minute apart.

- Hamstring exercise: Leg Curl—Bungee. Do 3 sets of 10, 1 minute apart.

DAY 12: CORE DAY III

Start with 2–3 minutes of stretching your quads.

Engage your core, as in Day 1.

- Quads exercise: Front Kick—Bungee. Do 3 sets of 10, 1 minute apart.

- Lower back exercise: Double-Arm Row—Bungee. Do 3 sets of 10, 1 minute apart.

DAY 13: CARDIO DAY

Exercise for no more than 30 minutes of "sprinted" cardio.

DAY 14: ABDOMEN/TRICEPS DAY

Start with 2–3 minutes of stretching your abdomen and triceps.

Engage your core, as in Day 1.

- Abdomen exercises: Leg Raise, Reverse Crunch. Do 10 of each, take a 1-minute break, then do 10 more of each. Do 3 sets.

- Triceps exercise: Overhead Extension—Bungee. Do 3 sets of 10, 1 minute apart.

DAY 15: OFF DAY

DAY 16: OFF DAY

DAY 17: CORE DAY I

Start with 2–3 minutes of stretching your shoulders.

Engage your core, as in Day 1.

- Abdomen exercises: Basic Crunch, Reverse Crunch, Side Crunch. Do 10 of each, take a 1-minute break, then do 10 more of each.

- Shoulder exercises: Bent Row—Bungee, Lateral Raise—Bungee, Straight-up Row—Bungee. Do 3 sets of 10, 1 minute apart.

DAY 18: EXTREMITIES DAY

Start with 5 minutes of stretching your biceps, triceps, and calves. Stretch each for 10 seconds with no break in between muscle groups. Repeat entire set 3 times.

Engage your core, as in Day 1.

- Biceps exercise: Alternating Curl—Bungee. Do 3 sets of 10, 1 minute apart.

- Triceps exercise: Bench or Chair Dip. Do 3 sets of 10, 1 minute apart.

- Calves exercise: Alternating Stair Raise. Do 3 sets of 10, 1 minute apart.

DAY 19: CORE DAY II

Start with 2–3 minutes of stretching your hamstrings.

Engage your core, as in Day 1.

- Glutes exercise: Adduction—Bungee. Do 3 sets of 10, 1 minute apart.

- Hamstring exercise: Reverse Hyperextension. Do 3 sets of 10, 1 minute apart.

DAY 20: CORE DAY III

Start with 2–3 minutes of stretching your quads.

Engage your core, as in Day 1.

- Quads exercise: Front Kick—Bungee. Do 3 sets of 10, 1 minute apart.

- Lower back exercise: Double-Arm Row—Bungee. Do 3 sets of 10, 1 minute apart.

DAY 21: CARDIO DAY

Exercise for more than 30 minutes of "sprinted" cardio.

DAY 22: ABDOMEN/TRICEPS DAY

Start with 2–3 minutes of stretching your abdomen and triceps.

Engage your core, as in Day 1.

- Abdomen exercises: Hip Thrust, Twisting Crunch. Do 10 of each, take a 1-minute break, then do 10 more of each.

- Triceps exercise: Nose Breaker, or Overhead Extension—Bungee. Do 3 sets of 10, 1 minute apart.

DAY 23: OFF DAY

DAY 24: OFF DAY

DAY 25: CORE DAY I

Start with 2–3 minutes of stretching your shoulders.

Engage your core, as in Day 1.

- Abdomen exercises: Basic Crunch, Leg Raise, Side Crunch. Do 3 sets of at least 10 or more (as many as you can do), 1 minute apart.

- Shoulder exercises: Bent Row—Bungee or Hand Weights, Front Raise—Bungee or Hand Weights, Lateral Raise—Bungee or Hand Weights. Do 3 sets of 10, 1 minute apart.

DAY 26: EXTREMITIES DAY

Start with 5 minutes of stretching your biceps, triceps, and calves. Stretch each for 10 seconds with no break in between muscle groups. Repeat entire set 3 times.

Engage your core, as in Day 1.

- Biceps exercise: Alternating Curl—Bungee. Do 3 sets of 10, 1 minute apart.

- Triceps exercise: Overhead Extension—Bungee. Do 3 sets of 10, 1 minute apart.

- Calves exercise: Standing Stair Raise. Do 3 sets of 10, 1 minute apart.

DAY 27: CORE DAY II

Start with 2–3 minutes of stretching your glutes.

Engage your core, as in Day 1.

- Glutes exercise: Adduction—Bungee. Do 3 sets of 10, 1 minute apart.

- Hamstring exercise: Leg Curl—Bungee. Do 3 sets of 10, 1 minute apart.

DAY 28: CORE DAY III

Start with 2–3 minutes of stretching your quads.

Engage your core, as in Day 1.

- Quads exercise: Front Kick—Bungee. Do 3 sets of 10, 1 minute apart.

- Lower back exercises: Double-Arm Row—Bungee. Do 3 sets of 10, 1 minute apart.

DAY 29: CARDIO DAY

Exercise for no more than 30 minutes of "sprinted" cardio.

DAY 30: ABDOMEN/TRICEPS DAY

Start with 2–3 minutes of stretching your abdomen and triceps.

Engage your core, as in Day 1.

- Abdomen exercises: Basic Crunch, Reverse Crunch. Do 10 of each, take a 1-minute break, then do 10 more of each.

- Triceps exercise: Bench or Chair Dip, or Overhead Two-Arm Extension—Hand Weights. Do 3 sets of 10, 1 minute apart.

DAY 31: OFF DAY

DAY 32: OFF DAY

MONITORING YOUR PROGRESS

Body shaping occurs gradually, so it can be very helpful to monitor your progress by measuring yourself at the beginning of your program and at the end of each week. If you do want to keep tabs as you transform yourself, this table should help.

MEASUREMENT	START	WEEK 1	WEEK 2	WEEK 3	WEEK 4
WEIGHT					
WAIST					
HIPS					
UPPER ARMS					

12.
FOUR-WEEK EXERCISE PLAN FOR THE HORMONE CATEGORY II—INTERMEDIATE/ADVANCED

WEEKLY CYCLE

DAY 1: CORE DAY I

Abdomen
Shoulders

DAY 2: EXTREMITIES DAY

Biceps
Triceps
Calves

DAY 3: CORE DAY II

Glutes
Hamstrings

DAY 4: CORE DAY III

Quads
Lower Back

DAY 5: CARDIO DAY

No more than 30 minutes of "sprinted" cardio

DAY 6: ABDOMEN/TRICEPS DAY

Abdomen

Triceps

DAY 7: OFF DAY

DAY 8: OFF DAY

FOUR-WEEK SCHEDULE

Once you've mastered these routines, you can mix them up with different selections from the exercises listed in chapter 8.

DAY 1: CORE DAY I

Start with 2–3 minutes of stretching your shoulders.

Sit on an armless chair, with back erect, shoulders back, heels flat against the floor, knees bent at 90 degrees, and hands on knees. You should be able to see your toes by simply looking down, without bending. You should also feel long, as if being pulled from the top of your head off your seat, as well as relaxed. Now gently pull your lower abdomen inward toward your back. Do not suck it in—*draw* your belly button into your back. Breathe normally. Hold this posture for 10 seconds. Repeat this 5 times.

You have now engaged your core and are ready to proceed with your Core Curriculum for today.

- Abdomen exercises: Basic Crunch, Reverse Crunch, Twisting Crunch. Do 10 of each, take a 1-minute break, then do 10 more of each.

- Shoulder exercises: Bent Row—Bungee or Hand Weights, Lateral Raise—Bungee or Hand Weights, Shoulder Press—Bungee or Hand Weights. Superset: Do a set of 10 of each exercise with no break. Rest 2 minutes and repeat. Do 3 supersets.

DAY 2: EXTREMITIES DAY

Start with 5 minutes of stretching your biceps, triceps, and calves. Stretch each for 10 seconds with no break in between muscle groups. Repeat entire set 3 times.

Engage your core, as in Day 1.

- Biceps exercises: Concentration Curl—Bungee, Alternating Curl—Bungee, Hammer Curl—Bungee. Superset: Do a set of 10 of each exercise without resting. Rest 2 minutes and repeat. Do 3 sets.

- Triceps exercise: Overhead Extension—Bungee, or Lying Extension—Hand Weights. Do 3 sets of 10, 1 minute apart.

- Calves exercise: Standing Stair Raise. Do 3 sets of 10 with a full range of motion, immediately followed by 10 half reps (top). Keep toes pointed inward (pigeon-toed).

DAY 3: CORE DAY II

Start with 2–3 minutes of stretching your hamstrings.

Engage your core, as in Day 1.

- Glutes exercise: Leg Curl—Bungee. Do 3 sets of 10, 1 minute apart.

- Hamstring exercises: Back Kick—Bungee, and Reverse Hyperextension. Do 3 sets of 10, 1 minute apart. Superset: Do a set of 10 of each exercise. Rest 2 minutes and repeat. Do 3 supersets.

DAY 4: CORE DAY III

Start with 2–3 minutes of stretching your quads.

Engage your core, as in Day 1.

- Quads exercise: Front Kick—Bungee. Do 3 sets of 10, 1 minute apart.

- Lower back exercise: Double-Arm Row—Bungee. Do 3 sets of 10, 1 minute apart. Use the heaviest cord resistance you can comfortably hold.

DAY 5: CARDIO DAY

Exercise for no more than 30 minutes of "sprinted" cardio.

DAY 6: ABDOMEN/TRICEPS DAY

Start with 2–3 minutes of stretching your abdomen and triceps.

Engage your core, as in Day 1.

- Abdomen exercises: Basic Crunch, Leg Raise. Do 10 of each, take a 1-minute break, then do 10 more of each.

- Triceps exercise: Overhead Extension—Bungee, or Lying Extension—Hand Weights. Do 10 with a full range of motion followed by 10 half reps (top). Rest 1 minute. Do 3 sets.

DAY 7: OFF DAY

DAY 8: OFF DAY

DAY 9: CORE DAY I

Start with 2–3 minutes of stretching your shoulders.

Engage your core, as in Day 1.

- Abdomen exercises: Basic Crunch, Hip Thrust, Side Crunch. Do 3 sets of as many as possible, 1 minute apart.

- Shoulder exercises: Bent Row—Bungee, Lateral Raise— Bungee, Straight-up Row—Bungee. Superset: Do a set of 10 of each exercise without resting. Rest 2 minutes and repeat. Do 3 supersets.

DAY 10: EXTREMITIES DAY

Start with 5 minutes of stretching your biceps, triceps, and calves. Stretch each for 10 seconds with no break in between muscle groups. Repeat entire set 3 times.

Engage your core, as in Day 1.

- Biceps exercise: Concentration Curl—Bungee, or Hammer Curl—Hand Weights. Do 3 sets of 10, 1 minute apart.

- Triceps exercise: Bench or Chair Dip, or Overhead Two-Arm Extension—Hand Weights. Do 3 sets of 10, 1 minute apart.

- Calves exercise: Stair Raise. Do 3 sets of 10, 1 minute apart. Circuit: Do a set of your choice of biceps and triceps exercises, followed by a set of Standing Stair Raises. Rest 2 minutes. Repeat for 3 circuits.

DAY 11: CORE DAY II

Start with 2–3 minutes of stretching your hamstrings.

Engage your core, as in Day 1.

- Glutes exercises: Adduction—Bungee, Back Kick—Bungee. Superset: Do a set of 10 of each exercise without resting. Rest 2 minutes and repeat. Do 3 supersets.

- Hamstring exercise: Leg Curl—Bungee. Do 3 sets of 10, 1 minute apart. Add ankle weights.

DAY 12: CORE DAY III

Start with 2–3 minutes of stretching your quads.

Engage your core, as in Day 1.

- Quads exercise: Front Kick—Bungee. Do 3 sets, with as many reps as possible per set, 1 minute apart.

- Lower back exercise: Double-Arm Row—Bungee. Do 3 sets of 10, 1 minute apart.

DAY 13: CARDIO DAY

Exercise for no more than 30 minutes of "sprinted" cardio.

THE BROWN FAT REVOLUTION EXERCISE PLAN

DAY 14: ABDOMEN/TRICEPS DAY

Start with 2–3 minutes of stretching your abdomen and triceps.

Engage your core, as in Day 1.

- Abdomen exercises: Leg Raise, Reverse Crunch. Superset: Do a set of 10 of each exercise. Rest 2 minutes and repeat. Do 3 supersets.

- Triceps exercise: Overhead Extension—Bungee. Do 3 sets of as many as possible in each set, 1 minute apart.

DAY 15: OFF DAY

DAY 16: OFF DAY

DAY 17: CORE DAY I

Start with 2–3 minutes of stretching your shoulders.

Engage your core, as in Day 1

- Abdomen exercises: Basic Crunch, Reverse Crunch, Side Crunch. Do 3 sets of as many possible, 1 minute apart.

- Shoulder exercises: Bent Row—Bungee, Lateral Raise—Bungee, Straight-up Row—Bungee. Superset: Do 10 reps of each exercise with no rest. Rest for 2 minutes. Do 3 supersets.

DAY 18: EXTREMITIES DAY

Start with 5 minutes of stretching your biceps, triceps, and calves. Stretch each for 10 seconds with no break in between muscle groups. Repeat entire set 3 times.

Engage your core, as in Day 1.

- Biceps exercise: Concentration Curl—Bungee, or Concentration Curl—Hand Weights. Do 10 with a full range of motion, then immediately do 10 half reps (top). Rest 1 minute and repeat. Do 3 sets.

- Triceps exercises: Nose Breaker, or Bench or Chair Dip; Overhead Extension—Bungee. Superset: Do a set of 10 of each exercise. Rest 2 minutes and repeat. Do 3 supersets.

- Calves exercise: Alternating Stair Raise. Do 3 sets of 10, 1 minute apart.

DAY 19: CORE DAY II

Start with 2–3 minutes of stretching your hamstrings.

Engage your core, as in Day 1.

- Glutes exercises: Adduction—Bungee, Back Kick—Bungee. Superset: Do a set of 10 of each exercise. Rest 2 minutes and repeat. Do 3 supersets.

- Hamstring exercise: Reverse Hyperextension. Do 3 sets of 10, 1 minute apart. Hold full extension for count of 20, then slowly release.

DAY 20: CORE DAY III

Start with 2–3 minutes of stretching your quads.

Engage your core, as in Day 1.

- Quads exercise: Front Kick—Bungee. Do 3 sets, 1 minute apart. Add ankle weights.

- Lower back exercise: Double-Arm Row—Bungee. Circuit: Do a set of 10 of each exercise without resting. Rest 2 minutes and repeat. Do 3 circuits.

DAY 21: CARDIO DAY

Exercise for no more than 30 minutes of "sprinted" cardio.

DAY 22: ABDOMEN/TRICEPS DAY

Start with 2–3 minutes of stretching your abdomen and triceps.

Engage your core, as in Day 1.

- Abdomen exercises: Basic Crunch, Reverse Crunch. Do 3 sets of as many as possible, 1 minute apart.

- Triceps exercises: Bench or Chair Dip, Overhead Extension—Bungee. Superset: Do a set of 10 reps of each exercise without resting. Rest 2 minutes and repeat. Do 3 supersets.

DAY 23: OFF DAY

DAY 24: OFF DAY

DAY 25: CORE DAY I

Start with 2–3 minutes of stretching your shoulders.

Engage your core, as in Day 1.

- Abdomen exercises: Basic Crunch, Leg Raise, Side Crunch. Do 3 sets of as many as possibly per set, 1 minute apart.

- Shoulder exercises: Bent Row—Bungee, Front Raise—Bungee, Lateral Raise—Bungee. Superset: Do a set of 10 reps of each exercise without resting. Rest 2 minutes and repeat. Do 3 supersets.

DAY 26: EXTREMITIES DAY

Start with 5 minutes of stretching your biceps, triceps, and calves. Stretch each for 10 seconds with no break in between muscle groups. Repeat entire set 3 times.

Engage your core, as in Day 1.

- Biceps exercise: Concentration Curl—Bungee, or Concentration Curl—Hand Weights. Pyramid: Do 10 reps with a heavy bungee cord. Immediately drop down to next resistance level, and do as many reps as you can to bring muscle to full fatigue. With hand weights, do 10 reps with a heavy weight, immediately drop it down to less weight, and do as many reps as you can to bring muscle to full fatigue.

- Triceps exercise: Overhead Extension—Bungee. Do 3 sets of 10, 1 minute apart.

- Calves exercise: Standing Stair Raise. Do 10 with feet together immediately followed by 10 with heels together, toes pointed out. Rest 1 minute. Do 3 sets.

DAY 27: CORE DAY II

Start with 2–3 minutes of stretching your glutes.

Engage your core, as in Day 1.

- Glutes exercises: Adduction—Bungee, Reverse Hyperextension. Superset: Do a set of 10 reps of each exercise without resting. Rest 2 minutes and repeat. Repeat for 3 supersets.

- Hamstring exercise: Leg Curl—Bungee. Do 3 sets of 10, 1 minute apart.

DAY 28: CORE DAY III

Start with 2–3 minutes of stretching your quads.

Engage your core, as in Day 1.

- Quads exercise: Front Kick—Bungee. Do 3 sets of as many as possible per set, 1 minute apart.

- Lower back exercise: Double-Arm Row—Bungee. Do 3 sets of 10, 1 minute apart.

DAY 29: CARDIO DAY

Exercise for no more than 30 minutes of "sprinted" cardio.

DAY 30: ABDOMEN/TRICEPS DAY

Start with 2–3 minutes of stretching your abdomen and triceps.

Engage your core, as in Day 1.

- Abdomen exercises: Hip Thrust, Reverse Crunch. Superset: Do a set of 10 of each exercise without resting. Rest 2 minutes and repeat. Do 3 sets.

- Triceps exercises: Kickback—Bungee or Hand Weights, or Overhead Extension—Bungee, Bench or Chair Dip. Superset: Do a set of 10 of each exercise without resting. Rest 2 minutes and repeat. Do 3 supersets.

DAY 31: OFF DAY

DAY 32: OFF DAY

MONITORING YOUR PROGRESS

Body shaping occurs gradually, so it can be very helpful to monitor your progress by measuring yourself at the beginning of your program and at the end of each week. If you do want to keep tabs as you transform yourself, this table should help.

MEASUREMENT	START	WEEK 1	WEEK 2	WEEK 3	WEEK 4
WEIGHT					
WAIST					
HIPS					
UPPER ARMS					

Appendix
THE BROWN FAT REVOLUTION SKIN CARE: YES, IT'S ALL ABOUT THE FAT!

Your skin is the biggest organ in your body, and its health is a direct reflection of your well-being. So you really do need to think of your skin as an organ that's as essential as your heart, lungs, or stomach.

But many of my patients as well as many other consumers instead treat their skin like the side of a house that's been painted without any underlying primer. Leave it exposed to the elements, and the damage will inevitably show up much more quickly. No skin-care regimen—and no makeup, no matter how beautiful—will make your skin look great if you don't take care of your underlying health first!

There are, unfortunately, inevitable changes to skin as you age, and those changes differ for everyone, due to many factors (genetics, oil content, smoking, sun exposure, stress, etc.), so there's no one-size-fits-all product or regimen that will work for all women. Maintaining your skin is a lifelong process; you must address what happens inside your body, such as hydration, hormonal balance, stress, bad eating habits that cause nutrients to be directed away from optimal skin restoration and repair, and the processing of toxins like alcohol or nicotine. Take care of yourself and it'll show. Don't take care of yourself and it'll show, too—but not in the way you want.

Everyone's skin is unique, because everyone is unique. Your skin is also unique at different times of the month, different times of your life, and in different environments. It reflects everything that's going on in your body and with your emotions, and will therefore be constantly in flux.

Don't allow yourself to get stuck in a skin-care rut the way so many women find themselves in a makeup rut. They use the same old thing because they know how to use it. It's comfortable. It's easy. But it's not working. And why should it, really, if they're still using the same products they first tried when they were in college, and now they're in their forties? Their lives have changed in the ensuing decades—and so has their skin.

Understanding your skin and having the best skin care possible will help enhance the visible effects once you have good brown fat back in your face.

BROWN FAT MEANS GOOD SKIN

My skin-care premise is simple: As your Eating and Exercise Plans transform your body while you get rid of old, wobbly yellow fat and make vast improvements in the consistency and distribution of your new, healthy brown fat, your skin is automatically going to plump up and look better. Young, dense brown fat fills out and supports your skin, adding the three-dimensional volume as well as the luster of youth to your face.

Obviously, the younger you are when you start replacing old yellow fat with new brown fat, the more quickly you'll get the volume back in your face. The sooner you do it, the less your skin falls, so it's easier to restore its original shape.

The word I like to use is "patina." For me, the best kind of skin patina is not flawless and wrinkle-free, but a surface that insinuates freshness and health. Ideally, what you want is skin with a glow to it. This means it has optimal hydration, an even tone (without blotchiness), a smooth texture (without large pores or acne), and a supportive understructure provided by good brown fat.

Even with a regular regimen of effective skin-care products, though, without a solid underpinning of good brown fat, trying to improve your skin is like trying to iron corduroy—it isn't going to happen.

SKIN FABRICS

As described in chapter 1, the skin on your face is placed atop several distinct pockets of fat. This skin is also made up of different "fabrics "on the same areas: your forehead, eye area, cheeks, and nose and central face.

Clearly, these fabrics are not identical. But I'll bet you treat them as if they were. And if you do, it might explain why you're unhappy with your current skin-care regimen.

When a plastic surgeon or dermatologist analyzes your face, he or she should approach each of the four areas differently. The thickness of your forehead is not the same as the thinness of your eyelids, for instance, and your cheeks have many more oil glands and a different thickness than your lips or chin.

In addition, the muscle action determining *how* these four fabrics move and age is not the same, either. How you kiss with, move, or purse your lips is not how you frown with your forehead or squint with your eyes when you've forgotten your sunglasses.

An easy way to think about your facial skin fabrics is by comparing them to the clothes you need to iron on laundry day. Some fabrics, like linen, need and can tolerate high heat; others, like silk, will burn in an instant with the wrong setting. So when I perform a laser treatment on a patient, if I didn't turn down the setting when I got near the eyelids, my patient would be in serious trouble. But if I didn't turn up the setting when working on the forehead or around the mouth, the laser would barely be effective.

In other words, what's more important than the product itself is the *application* of the product. You don't need four separate products for your four different skin fabrics, but you do need to use a different application to different parts of the face, progressing from areas where you need the most help to areas where you need the least.

For example, you should apply moisturizer first on the lower eyelids, followed by your forehead, temples, cheekbone area, and central facial area. For an exfoliant, use it first on your forehead, then move down to your chin, cheek, nose, and around your mouth, but not on the lower or upper eyelids.

Ask yourself what needs treatment with that specific product, and use it only where it's needed.

BASIC SKIN-CARE REGIMEN

Whether you are in Hormone Category I or Hormone Category II, you will need few products to keep your skin glowing. Here are your regimen basics.

Note: If you have any skin issues (acne, age spots, blotchiness, discoloration or hyperpigmentation, dullness, rosacea, etc.), you should consult a dermatologist for advice.

MORNING AND EVENING SKIN CARE
Morning Skin Care

1. Cleanse (optional)

2. Treat (if needed)

3. Moisturize/protect (sunscreen is not optional!)

Evening Skin Care

1. Cleanse

2. Exfoliate with Retin-A (if needed, as prescribed by your plastic surgeon or dermatologist)

3. Treat (if needed)

4. Moisturize

ABOUT CLEANSERS

The goal of a good cleansing is to restore, not irritate skin. The only way to do that is with a gentle cleanser. And to tell you the truth, understanding the thousands of cleansers on the market is actually extremely simple. They're either mild, or they aren't. That's it! Any other claims are specious at best.

Most cleansers just remove dirt, while some remove oil as well. So unless you have extremely oily skin, all you need is a gentle, soap-free, *nonabrasive* cleanser to wash away the dirt.

Unfortunately, I've seen countless patients over the years who think they have skin problems when all they have is what I call Overwashing Syndrome, thinking that they need to have squeaky-clean skin. In fact, most women do not need to wash their faces twice a day. Sure, you can if you want to, and you certainly need to wash well at night to remove the grime of the day, but your face is not going to somehow become magically filthy overnight if all you do is moisturize before bed and then go to sleep! Even if you have acne, too much washing will remove the acid mantle and protective lipids from your skin, allowing the bacteria that causes acne to multiply, so your skin will actually get worse.

Many of my patients with dry skin like to wash their skin with a cleansing oil. It doesn't make your skin greasy; instead, it hydrates as it cleanses, and maintains and protects your skin's acid mantle.

ABOUT EXFOLIATION

Exfoliation is one of those techniques in skin care that, like hydration, has pretty much immediate results—but it's also not understood very well. Exfoliating doesn't mean that you need to rub your face raw with grainy grit.

Each cell in your body has a finite lifespan, and skin cells are no different. For everyone, cell turnover decreases with age.

As skin cells start to age, they slowly move from the deeper layers of skin toward the surface, called the stratum corneum, where they're sloughed off on a daily basis. In other words, exfoliation is just a way to help you get rid of dead skin.

The problem with dead skin cells is that they get sticky, and if not sloughed off well, your skin looks dull and blah. Exfoliators break up the connections between these sticky cells, allowing them to come off easily.

There are many different levels of exfoliators, from very mild over-the-counter (OTC) creams to much more intense products. I'm not a big believer in anything but the mildest OTC exfoliators, because consumers tend to get out of control when using them and do too much, too fast. This often leads to irritation, blotchiness, and redness, and a potentially long healing period.

Here are a few tips.

The exfoliation process is directly affected by your environment, so you need to adjust how often you exfoliate depending on the time of year and the humidity level. In very dry winter environments, for instance, you'll probably need to exfoliate less often, as the air is dry and your skin cells will be less sticky, so they'll slough off more easily.

Home microdermabrasion kits can be terrifically effective, but you must follow the directions carefully. Start out very slowly to avoid irritation. If the directions say to use only once or twice a week at first, that does not mean every other day!

Prescription exfoliators, such as Retin-A, must also be used scrupulously according to directions. I'll tell my patients to use it on Monday, Wednesday, and Friday, with the weekends off. Instead, they'll use it every night, and then call me to say, "My face is red and burning. Help!"

ABOUT MOISTURIZERS

Even dermatologists can't agree about how best to use moisturizers. Some studies in the medical literature maintain that moisturizing the skin decreases irritation and protects the skin from environmental pollutants, while others claim that long-term moisturizing actually *increases* irritation. (Actually, it's probably specific ingredients in different moisturizers that account for these disagreements.)

Moisturizers usually contain occlusive compounds, such as petroleum, to prevent water loss; humectants, which are compounds that attract water, such as glycerol; and emollients, which don't add hydration but are used as a filler to improve the "glide" of the product.

No wonder consumers are confused—which means they often waste huge amounts of money on the latest cream to get the big bad hype machine behind it.

The bottom line about moisturizers is that *not one* has been scientifically shown to improve skin quality and appearance. The reason is simple: Moisturizers are not treatment creams. They have no druglike properties. They can't reduce wrinkles, but they can plump up your skin's appearance by holding in moisture and creating a barrier between your skin cells and the stresses of the environment.

And as oil production decreases with age, many women find that their skin becomes progressively drier. Working and living in rooms with low humidity doesn't help. So feel free to use a good moisturizer—but bear in mind that there are absolutely *no* ingredients in moisturizers that warrant a huge price tag!

SKIN-CARE INGREDIENTS THAT WORK

Besides tackling your fat from the inside out, you can address your skin from the outside in. While there is no skin cream that can magically erase decades of life from your skin, there are many products containing ingredients that can greatly enhance your skin's appearance, texture, and tone.

But because there are thousands of OTC products from which to choose—some costing next to nothing and some costing hundreds of dollars—you'll need to decipher the language of what's effective and what's little more than effective hype. If you read the ingredient lists, which by law must be on the box, you will see a bewildering smattering of complicated chemical names you can barely pronounce, much less figure out.

Good products do what they say they're going to do (not more, and not less).

Products that really do work are cleansers, sunscreens, basic hydrating moisturizers, exfoliators, and lighteners/brighteners. That said, there are very few active ingredients in OTC skin-care products that have been *scientifically* shown to work. Only one prescription ingredient, retinoic acid, has been FDA approved for use on fine lines and wrinkles. No OTC wrinkle cream can make that claim.

ALPHA HYDROXY ACID (AHA)

Hear the word "acid" and you tend to think of something that burns, but the kind of acids used on skin can improve its appearance, by working as an exfoliator or by helping to reduce discoloration.

AHAs (glycolic acid, lactic acid, malic acid, alpha hydroxyethanoic acid, alpha hydroxyoctanoic acid, alpha hydroxylcaprylic acid, hydroxycaproic acid, citric acid, and hydroxyl fruit acids) are all good exfoliators. The concentration can go up to 10 percent in OTC creams; 10–40 percent concentrations can be used by trained skin-care professionals (nurses, medical aestheticians in spas and salons); and concentrations over 40 percent can be used only by medical doctors. These higher concentrations can have good results in repairing skin's elastic fibers as well as stimulating collagen growth, but the higher the percentage, the higher the risk of overdoing it, so consulting an experienced physician or plastic surgeon is a must.

ALPHA LIPOIC ACID (ALA)

Alpha lipoic acid is a scavenger for reactive oxygen particles (free radicals that damage your skin), and has been shown to increase collagen synthesis in the skin of rats. Although similar studies on human skin weren't quite as statistically effective, patients tested were happy with the results and saw visible improvement.

HYDROQUINONE

Hydroquinone is a bleaching agent that's used in low doses in OTC lightening or brightening products. It helps fade age or sun spots, discoloration from blemishes, and freckles. These products won't alter your skin's color, but can help to even out its overall tone.

Many dermatologists consider hydroquinone to be the best skin-lightening agent available. In OTC products, the concentration can be no more than 2 percent. Concentrations up to 5 percent are available by prescription.

Although the FDA has approved hydroquinone as safe and effective, it is not available in any OTC products (only by prescription) in some countries in Europe and Asia, for fears that it may possibly cause liver damage or increase the risk of cancer. But the studies that came to these conclusions looked at hydroquinone taken *orally* in extremely high concentrations. Unfortunately, these findings have been distorted in the media. Perhaps one of the problems is that, as with exfoliators, consumers tend not to follow directions and can overuse it, causing irritation and redness.

RETINOIC ACID/TRETINOIN

Retinoic acid (the acid form of vitamin A) is a potent and natural skin antioxidant. Applied topically, it will improve the appearance of the skin, as it can visibly diminish fine wrinkles and improve pigmentation. Retinoic acid is available only in very low concentrations OTC, in the form of retinaldehyde, retinol, and retinol esters. Retinols have been extensively studied and are effective in improving skin; retinol esters show promise but have yet to be proved to be effective at the scientific level.

But I think it is much better to see a dermatologist or plastic surgeon, as that is the only way to get prescription-strength retinoic acid (or tretinoin), the active ingredient in the formulations called Retin-A and Renova.

In higher concentrations, retinoic acid is the only effective wrinkle-fighting ingredient that has been approved by the FDA; it has been shown to increase collagen synthesis as well as the skin's fibroblast cells (the cells that produce collagen), and can dramatically improve dyschromia (hyperpigmentation, or age spots) and fine wrinkles. It can be a truly remarkable rejuvenator. But—and this is a big but!—the reason Retin-A and Renova are available only by prescription is that they have the potential to cause intense irritation.

Because many consumers know that Retin-A and Renova are FDA approved and are effective, they are eager to use them. Or perhaps I should say *over*eager. Far too many women think Retin-A and Renova are magic potions and not only use them way too much, but use them on their own instead of within the context of an entire skin-care regimen.

If you are prescribed Retin-A or Renova, you must follow the instructions of your dermatologist or plastic surgeon, or your face can become red and irritated. Do not overdo it! There are different formulas and concentrations to help minimize any redness, and it's common to have to try different levels to find the one that works the best for you. Bear in mind that sunscreen is an absolute must as a daily commitment, because tretinoin makes your skin much more susceptible to severe sunburn.

VITAMIN C

Vitamin C, or L-ascorbic acid, is commonly used in many OTC anti-aging formulations. It has been shown to be effective in the deeper levels of skin, notably on the intercellular space to reorganize collagen and stimulate the production of elastic fibers, as well as on the surface as a potent antioxidant.

USE YOUR SUNSCREEN

I'd say the tipping point for complaints about skin come for women in the middle of the Hormone Category I years. These patients usually tell me two things the minute they sit down: "I hate my skin," and "I look old."

For them, the dazzle is gone and the wrinkles are not.

Obviously, I need these patients to be more specific about their concerns, so I make them do something they usually don't want to do—pick up a mirror and talk about what precisely they see, and what precisely bothers them the most.

And then I tell them that the single most important product they can use for skin rejuvenation is sunscreen.

Do they listen? Not always—too many women are still addicted to tanning. Some of them have tans that stun me, as they look like a Louis Vuitton suitcase. But then I tell them that if they don't use sunscreen, particularly after a long and/or costly procedure, it's like a dentist putting veneers on a patient who doesn't brush her teeth. They might as well throw their money out the window. (This is especially true with certain kinds of laser procedures, which are extremely effective at getting rid of hyperpigmentation, or brown spots, as well as rejuvenating skin, but which often need several sessions to complete. It's a process that takes some time—but after just one afternoon unprotected in the sun, you're back to square one.)

But wearing sunscreen isn't just about saving money—it's probably the most important prerequisite for healthy, young skin. The cumulative effect of a lifetime of sun exposure damages the layers of your skin, alters its DNA, and can lead to deadly skin cancers. And it's not just summertime tanning on the beach that causes damage; incidental, chronic, daily sun exposure wreaks even more havoc. I see this on the faces I treat—the left side is always more damaged because of its increased exposure to the sun while driving.

The bottom line is that if you're trying to improve your health and your appearance, get over the sun. For me, the sun and cigarettes are like the worst of all possible worlds—they just destroy everything.

Getting into the daily sunscreen habit is *much* easier than changing the way you eat or starting a regular exercise routine. It takes barely a minute a day to apply sunscreen each morning, and then again if you're going out in the sun during the day. And it's guaranteed to work, making it by far the most inexpensive and quickest improvement you can make for your skin.

Here are a few tips.

Get into the habit of putting sunscreen on in the morning, after you brush your teeth. It needs at least twenty to thirty minutes to activate, so if you put it on just before you leave the house, you won't have any protection right away.

You don't need to use a moisturizer and a sunscreen in the morning, as that can make your skin too greasy. Choose either a sunscreen intended for use on the face, or a good moisturizer with a high SPF (sun protection factor).

Some of my patients have told me that they don't like using sunscreen because the brands they've tried are thick and make their skin sweaty. Fortunately, most sunscreens are not expensive, so if you buy a brand you don't like, use it on the rest of your body so it doesn't go to waste, and find another one that feels good on your face. Like all skin-care products, how different sunscreens feel and smell is highly subjective.

One of the biggest problems with sunscreen is that consumers don't use enough. This can have dire consequences, since sunscreen SPFs are tested using the proper amount; use less and you won't be getting the SPF you think you are. Usually, at least a teaspoon of sunscreen is recommended just for the face. Measure it out and you'll likely be surprised at how much it is.

SPF measures only protection against UVB radiation, or the sun's burning rays. Ingredients to look for are titanium dioxide, avobenzone, and micronized zinc, and the minimum SPF should be 15. I usually recommend using an SPF of at least 30. SPF does not measure against UVA rays, which are the kind that cause aging and wrinkles. Look for sunscreens that are "broad-spectrum," as they should have UVA protection as well.

Get into the habit of seeing a dermatologist on a regular basis—at least once a year—for a full-body check of moles and age spots. If you notice any changes to preexisting moles, you must consult a dermatologist immediately, as this is one possible indication of skin cancer.

SKIN-CARE MYTHS

While visiting a department store with my wife recently, I was absolutely flabbergasted at the bewildering array of products in the cosmetics department. My wife went off to browse, and I sat down on a bench to watch shoppers enter this skin-care paradise.

It was a very entertaining yet sobering experience. Entertaining because many of the men and women working the counters were consummate professionals. They knew how to explain skin care, how to answer their customers' questions, and how to sell while creating a memorable, pampering experience.

But some of the salespeople got it all wrong. They hyped ineffective ingredients, didn't offer products meeting the customers' needs, misdiagnosed common skin conditions (which can be dangerous), and created regimens with many different products that were clearly not designed to follow one another in a cohesive program. And I watched their customers lap it up.

Many of these consumers had fallen for the potent power of skin-care myths. So let's take a look at some of the most common of these.

YOU CAN SELF-DIAGNOSE YOUR SKIN-CARE ISSUES

If you have any questions about your skin, you should get advice *only* from a competent, board-certified dermatologist or plastic surgeon. No matter how many skin-care books, articles, or Web sites you read—and no matter how good they are (and many of these sources are extremely well written and soundly informative)—the average consumer is still not a medical professional and as such is just not capable of making an informed diagnosis. Self-diagnosis is particularly dangerous if you have moles or any new skin conditions, and think you have a simple irritation or pimple when in fact you have a melanoma that can kill you.

Yet far too many of my patients have told me that they get their skin-care advice not from a dermatologist or a plastic surgeon, but from a salesperson at the cosmetic counter, or from an article or two, or from their friends. Well, as I said already, the salespeople might be terrific, or they might be dead wrong. Advertising-dependent articles might have a slant you don't know about. And friends might mean well and love a certain product that works wonders for them, but your skin might need something completely different.

You owe it to your skin—and your life—to get the best possible advice about your skin.

IF YOUR SKIN-CARE CREAM ISN'T WORKING RIGHT AWAY, IT'S NOT GOING TO WORK AT ALL

One of the reasons why the skin-care business is such big business is because consumers are extremely fickle. They get a new product, try it, don't see results, don't stick with it because they don't get what they're hoping for right away, and then move on to the next product in an endless cycle of frustration and worsening skin.

But for skin-care products, you need patience. Few consumers understand that any product, even if it doesn't have active drug ingredients, needs time to become effective. Even basic hydration from a simple OTC moisturizer will not happen overnight. And products with any sort of potent treatment usually take at least six to eight weeks to become effective. That's up to two months!

The other thing you must do is follow instructions. If the box says "Use sparingly," that is not giving you license to slather on the product. An OTC product doesn't need a prescription, but it can still contain ingredients that have a druglike effect on your skin. Using more of this product than absolutely necessary can cause your skin to react with irritation, redness, swelling, breakouts, or blotchiness.

Remember, you have four different skin fabrics on your face, so treat only one at a time! Don't try to minimize forehead wrinkles, lessen crepey eyelid skin, and smooth your cheeks all at once.

MORE PRODUCTS = BETTER SKIN

Not only do many consumers overuse the products they have, they use far too many of these products.

You should treat your skin the same way an allergist treats a patient who's sensitive to certain foods. Start with the very basics, and gradually add on. That way, you won't overload your system, and you'll be able to identify any ingredients that might not be right for you.

For example, fragrance is an ingredient that is a common allergen. So while you might love the smell of a particular cream, the fragrance in that cream might trigger redness or flakiness.

Nor should you layer on a toner, serum, moisturizer, wrinkle cream, and treatment cream, even if your skin reacts to these products individually. That's way too much stuff on your face! Less is more. All you need is skin that is clean, hydrated, sun-protected during the day, and, perhaps, treated according to your dermatologist's or plastic surgeon's suggestions. That's it.

A MOISTURIZER CAN GET RID OF YOUR WRINKLES

As I already discussed in the section on moisturizers, one of the biggest skin-care myths is that a moisturizer can reduce wrinkles, because that's what so many of the ads imply.

It's worth repeating here that moisturizers do work. At *moisturizing*. Many of them contain humectants that can literally draw water into the skin. So wouldn't it follow that if our skin is more moist, it might be less wrinkled? Perhaps, but that notion gets distorted and extrapolated way too much into the erroneous belief that the wrinkle is going to go away. A good moisturizer is not an antiwrinkle cream. What it does is protect your skin from not getting any worse, but it will never repair a wrinkle that already exists.

What OTC ingredients can do is improve your skin's appearance. The best of them might be able to give the optical illusion of wrinkle disappearance, but the wrinkle is still there.

Furthermore, if an OTC product claims to have penetrated down to the lower levels of your skin to make changes where wrinkles start to form, they are very likely heading into the realm of exaggeration. Only prescription drugs can penetrate skin layers.

IF THERE'S SOMETHING WRONG WITH YOUR SKIN, IT MEANS YOUR SKIN-CARE PRODUCTS AREN'T WORKING

Skin, being the largest organ of your body, doesn't exist in a vacuum. What I tell my patients is that skin is just not the whole deal. It's only part of the deal—and part of your overall health picture.

As a result, one of the reasons why so many women are disappointed with their skin-care products is that there are other issues going on besides skin. So even if your skin-care product works as intended, and is a terrific product, it's not capable of removing your jowls, or erasing your wrinkles, or filling out your face the way good brown fat can.

Instead of being disappointed with your product, you should realize that if there's to be any disappointment, it's with unrealistic expectations.

YOUTHFUL SKIN MEANS FLAWLESS SKIN

I've seen the skin on some Hollywood stars—you know the kind I mean. Skin that is so freakishly smooth on a woman in her forties or fifties that you can't stop staring, and not for the right reasons. But if you can't tear your eyes off a face that no longer resembles anything real, or that's in possession of a forehead that doesn't move when the lips are smiling, there's no possibility of this face being thought of as youthful or vibrant or stunning. This is not a look to aspire to.

If you were Rembrandt, and about to paint a woman's face, even a woman who's forty-five years old, would you make her skin flawlessly smooth? Would it diminish from her beauty if she were not flawless? Of course not!

Unfortunately, I think it's an uphill battle convincing women that an ideal beauty is *not* one with allegedly flawless, preternaturally smooth and super-plump skin, especially on women of a certain age. (And that it is particularly noticeable when the face is scary smooth while the rest of the body, especially the neck and hands, is not.) Certainly, when used judiciously, injectible fillers and Botox can greatly enhance many different faces. But so can good brown fat!

You can have beautiful, youthful skin by doing nothing more than following the Eating and Exercise Plans in this book, and adding a simple yet effective skin-care regimen that addresses your unique needs.

YOU DON'T NEED A GOOD SKIN-CARE REGIMEN—QUICK FIXES WILL DO THE TRICK

The kind of patient I won't treat is the kind of patient who shows up demanding some of the most aggressive skin-care procedures, such as chemical peels or laser therapy, yet refuses to accept that they also—and will always—need a daily, meaningful, consistent skin-care program. Without a regular regimen, it's like thinking you can speak Italian in Rome when all you know is how to order espresso at a café in Brooklyn. Without a proper amount of time spent learning the basics, the advanced work just isn't going to happen.

Having intensive or invasive procedures is not an excuse to cover up a poor-quality lifestyle. For instance, many of my patients who are fond of spending a lot of time on the beach want a total facial CO_2 laser resurfacing, which is highly effective at undoing sun damage but is a highly aggressive procedure. It's also painful, with a long recuperation period, during which you can absolutely not go in the sun. Or smoke. Yet these patients are chain-smoking tanaholics who want a quick fix now, rather than a slower program that might help them undo their bad habits. They want me to do the work for them, but they're not willing to do the work themselves to stop the damage from happening in the first place!

Treat your skin with the respect and care it deserves. A very small amount of daily attention will keep it healthy and glowing through the rest of your life.

INDEX